Spinal Stabilization
The New Science of Back Pain

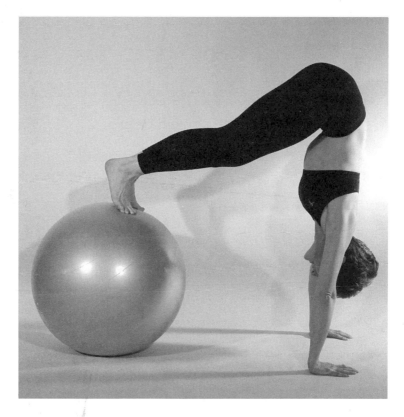

Effective solutions for people with low back pain

Effective conditioning for competitive athletes

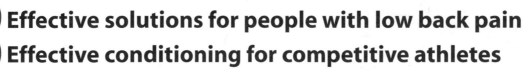

The new approach used by rehabilitation experts and top sports conditioning coaches.
Discover how *spinal stabilization* can control your back pain and improve your performance in any sport!

Jemmett, Richard S., 1961 -
Spinal Stabilization - The New Science of Back Pain

ISBN   0 - 9688715 - 0 - X

Proof Reader: Meagan B.L. Jemmett
Photography: Rick Jemmett
Anatomy Illustrations: Margaret Galloway
Models: Chris Bridge, Sarah Gordon, Margot Jemmett, Rosalind Rossi
Printed By: etc. Press Ltd., Halifax, Canada

Distributed by:

OPTP *The Conservative Care Specialists*
. . . .
PO Box 47009, Minneapolis, MN 55447
(800) 367-7393   (763) 553-0452

Lawyer's Contribution:
Medical knowledge is updated regularly. As new information becomes available, changes to treatment guidelines and
the management of various medical conditions are inevitable. The author and publisher have taken great care to
ensure that the information presented is accurate, up-to-date and in keeping with the highest standard of care at the
time of publication. However, readers are strongly encouraged to consult with their licensed health care professional to
confirm that the information contained in this book meets with the latest standards of practice. The author and
publisher are not responsible for errors or omissions or for any consequences which may arise from application of the
information in this book.

Acknowledgements

I would like to sincerely thank my wife Margot and daughter Meagan who have made it possible for me to write this book. Their willingness to sacrifice their own time and too much of our time as a family were instrumental in helping this project reach completion. Meagan, your editing and proofreading talents are so greatly appreciated (despite your sometimes brutal treatment of my attempts at narrative). Margot, your humour, personal resolve and physical strength continue to impress and amaze me.

For their support (and tolerance), many thanks to my colleagues at Maritime Physiotherapy, especially Robert MacDonald, David MacDonald and Sarah Gordon, and of course the many patients and conditioning clients whose motivation and willingness to try something new provided me with an ongoing source of confidence in this project. Thanks specifically to Bep, Bruce, Debbie, Maggie, Chris and Anne Marie for your contributions to this book.

For their inspiration and demonstration of what it is to be a professional, a clinician and an educator, my thanks to Anne Augur, Sharon Shafir and Molly Verrier at the University of Toronto.

For their inspiration and demonstration of what it is to be a friend, my gratitude to Mike Drinkwater, Nola and Mathew Hart, Rob MacDonald and Evelyn Sutton, and Simon Roberts.

Finally, a book of this type could not be conceived of let alone written for 'public consumption' without the scientific research conducted by a variety of professionals from around the world. I would like to single out the following for their substantial contributions to the rehabilitation of people who have orthopaedic pathology: Diane Lee, Stuart McGill, Carolyn Richardson, Gwendolen Jull, Paul Hodges, Julie Hides and Manohar Panjabi. My ability to effectively treat people with spinal conditions has been enhanced tremendously thanks to the research generated by these individuals. This book is merely a reconstruction of their work in a language I hope the non-medical professional can understand.

Rick Jemmett

Spinal Stabilization
The New Science of Back Pain

Introduction

This is a book for people like you who have a back.

It is a book for people who have back pain and for people who would rather avoid the experience of back pain altogether. It is a book for people - nurses, parents, lawyers and labourers, butchers, bakers and software makers - who need a healthy back to do their jobs and everyday activities. It is a book for people who run, ride, swim or skate; who throw things, swing things, paddle things or kick things - and who want to avoid injury and improve their athletic performance.

Spinal Stabilization is a new concept in rehabilitation and sports conditioning based on up-to-date scientific research into the anatomy and mechanical behaviour of our spine and its supporting muscles. This important new research - *the new science of back pain* - has led to a vastly improved understanding of how our back is supposed to work. With this new knowledge physical therapists in Australia and Canada have developed an exciting and unique approach to designing conditioning programs for athletes and rehabilitation programs for people with back injuries. This new, science-based approach is already being used by enlightened physical therapists and elite-level sport conditioning coaches across North America.

Spinal Stabilization

Rehabilitation professionals have always known that in order to have a healthy back, a person must have strong abdominal and spinal muscles. For decades, physical therapists and doctors have prescribed back and abdominal exercises for their patients with back pain. The trouble was, many patients with back pain didn't seem to get much better using standard sit-ups and back strengthening exercises. In fact, some people felt their back and neck pain became even worse with these exercises. As it turned out, these exercise prescriptions were limited by a lack of knowledge; rehabilitation professionals didn't yet know enough about the specific function of the spine and its muscles to design consistently successful exercise programs for people with back or spinal pathology.

Similarly, coaches and athletes have long relied on the abdominal and back strengthening exercises which originated in the body-building world. While these exercises are useful in developing the large, power generating muscles of the trunk, they do little to train the deeper muscles of the abdomen and back. These deep spinal muscles - sometimes referred to as core muscles - are critical to achieving optimal performance in virtually all sports. In fact, they are critical to ideal spine function in all activities.

The New Science of Back Pain

Over the past few years, researchers in Canada, the United States, Japan and Australia have shed new light on the way our spine works. Thus, the *spinal stabilization* approach is based on a dramatically improved understanding of the function of the spinal column and its muscles.

We now know that the various muscles of the spine serve very different purposes: some act as *position sensors*, some act as *stabilizers* and others work to create *powerful* movements. With this improved understanding of spinal function, we have been able to develop more effective exercise prescriptions which train the various trunk muscles for their specific functions.

While virtually all people with back pain will benefit from the spinal stabilization method, it is important to realize that not all of the exercises described in this book will be appropriate for everyone. Different people with different types of back problems at different points in their recovery process will be best served by a program designed for their specific circumstances. Therefore, if you have back pain, you are strongly encouraged to consult with a licensed physical therapist who uses this approach in their daily practice. He or she will be able to select the safest and most effective combination of exercises for you and your back problem.

For those of you who are recreational or competitive athletes and would like a more high-performance, injury-resistant spine, you too will find plenty to work with in this book. In fact, some of the more advanced exercises will challenge even olympic-level athletes. Even though you may not have selected this book to solve a back pain problem, consultation with a physical therapist may still be beneficial in terms of selecting the most appropriate exercises for your sport and ensuring that you are using good technique.

The Why and How of Spinal Stabilization

In our daily work with patients and athletes, physical therapists have learned that people are most likely to carry through with their exercise program if they understand the why and how of their rehabilitation.

The 'why' refers to why it is that their back hurts and the 'how' refers to how it is that our exercise prescription will help them. In order to understand back injury, one must first have a basic understanding of how the spine is built and how it works. Therefore, we will begin in chapter one with a brief look at the anatomy and function of the spinal column.

The second chapter looks at the medical terminology used to define different types of back problems. Diagnostic terms like 'spondylosis', 'sciatica' and 'degenerative disc disease' will be explained in everyday language helping you to better understand your back problem. Chapter two will also discuss the extent to which stabilization training can be expected to benefit people with these different diagnoses. Thus chapters one and two will help you to understand the *why* of back pain rehabilitation.

Chapter three describes in detail the various concepts which form the foundation of a stabilization-based exercise program. These concepts are critical to your success with this approach so special attention should be paid to this section. This is true whether you are recovering from back injury, managing a chronic spinal condition or improving your core strength for sport performance reasons. Therefore, chapter three is concerned with the 'how' of stabilization training.

Chapters four, five and six will teach you how to apply the principles of stabilization training. Pictures and descriptions of all the exercises are included in these sections. You will learn how to do the exercises correctly and how to move from beginner to more advanced variations safely. These chapters discuss the use of stabilization training for people with back pain, the role of stabilization-based exercises in back injury prevention programs, and the ability of stabilization training to improve athletic performance.

Before we go any further, lets deal with a question many readers probably have on their minds at this point. What is meant by spinal stability and why is it so important?

Stability - The Key to Healthy Movement

Our spinal column is a series of 25 separate spinal bones called *vertebrae* connected by soft tissues known as *ligaments* and the spinal *discs* which attach one vertebrae to the next. The linking together of all these bones produces a flexible column which allows us the freedom to move in many directions. However, recent research reminds us that this flexibility comes at a price.

The spinal column (the vertebrae, discs and ligaments) is a relatively weak structure. In fact, an adult spinal column will collapse with as little as nine pounds of weight applied to it. This means that without muscles our spine would not be able to support even our own body weight. Without muscle, the joints of the spinal column would not remain *stable*.

The extent to which stability is important for a healthy back can be a difficult concept for people to come to terms with. This may be due to people's tendency to confuse joint stability with muscular flexibility. Indeed, many people seem to think that an increase in joint stability must come at the expense of their flexibility. This is definitely not the case. Joint stability refers to the ability of a joint to move freely and fully while also remaining properly aligned. Flexibility, while certainly a good thing, has more to do with the 'stretchiness' of our muscles than it does the *sureness* or *integrity of fit* of a spinal joint.

All joints, spinal as well as shoulder, knee, ankle and others, need to be free to move through their normal range of motion while maintaining a solid, correct fit between the parts of the bones which make up the joint. If this fit becomes too 'loose' the joint will begin to function incorrectly, usually with pain being the first indication of a problem.

When is a painful back like a damaged door hinge ...?

For years I tried to come up with a good analogy to help patients understand these concepts. Oddly enough, my daughter provided me with what I had been looking for. One day when Meagan was about eleven, I noticed that the door to her room was sagging on its hinges and dragging its leading edge on the floor as it opened or closed. On closer inspection I could see that the top hinge had recently been ripped off the door frame and then carefully put back in place. The screws which had held the top hinge to the door frame had of course been pulled out, leaving the holes too large and ragged to hold the original screws firmly. The hinge, in other words, had lost its correct fit and stability. Even though 'someone' had managed to get the hinge back in place and the door working, eventually the hinge started to pull away from the frame. Within a few days the door wouldn't open or close properly.

In a simple way, joints in our body are like hinges on a door. The two bones which form a joint fit together in a precise way just as the two halves of the hinge must fit together in order for the door to open and close smoothly. In the case of a door hinge, this fit or stability is simply dependent on the screws which anchor the hinge to the edge of the door. In our body, spinal joint stability is much more complicated.

Spinal joint stability is dependent on healthy ligaments and spinal discs, correct muscle function and the ability of our brain to coordinate dozens of spinal muscles in a continuous fashion while our body moves. Joint stability can be lost instantly in the case of a severe injury. These instabilities may also develop slowly, due to normal wear and tear on joints, certain types of athletic training or even habitually poor posture.

When spinal joint stability is lost, a variety of structures in the spine may suffer the consequences. In the case of my daughter's door, the hinges would have been exposed to some abnormal wear and tear as would the bottom of the door as it dragged on the floor. In a similar way, the spinal joints, discs or ligaments might be forced to tolerate unusual loads resulting in pain. The spinal nerve roots which pass between the bones of the spine might even be compressed, resulting in both back and leg pain. Spinal stability is therefore important in ensuring that our spine works correctly from a mechanical perspective, minimizing our risk of pain and potential disability.

Aside from pain and injury issues, a stable spine is also a more high-performance spine. For both recreational and competitive athletes, spinal stabilization training will increase power development through the arms, legs and trunk while lowering the risk of 'overuse' injuries. Virtually all athletes will realize sport performance improvements as well as a lower risk of low back injury and pain.

Perhaps most importantly, spinal stabilization training is actually enjoyable. The exercises, especially those utilizing the 'SwissBall' or 'StabilityBall', make exercise seem like play. Patients and clients alike report a much higher degree of satisfaction with their 'new' programs in part because spinal stabilization training works well but also because they begin to sincerely look forward to their exercise sessions ... try finding someone who can say that about traditional abdominal training!

Thank you for choosing this book and taking the first step toward incorporating spinal stabilization training into your daily routine. Please read all of the text - chapters one, two and three - before beginning the exercises. At all times use caution recognizing that, as with any exercise program, exercises done incorrectly will at best be ineffective but at worst may cause injury.

If you have any kind of back pain, any neck, shoulder, hip or knee problems, balance disorders or any other medical condition which could possibly be made worse with exercise, you must consult with a physician, physical therapist or chiropractor before beginning these exercises.

Chapter 1
Spinal Anatomy & Function: How your back works

Basic Anatomy of the Spine

When teaching patients about how their back is built and how it works, I have found it helpful to describe the back as a structure consisting of three layers. Each of these three layers - the deep, the middle and the outer - has a specific role to play in overall spine function.

The deep layer is made up of the 25 bones or *vertebrae* which form the spine along with the spinal discs which attach one vertebrae to the next. This deep layer also includes a variety of ligaments which are attached to the sides, front, and back of the vertebrae. The final component of the deep layer is a series of tiny muscles which run from one vertebrae to the next. These deep muscles and ligaments span the entire length of the spinal column, from your neck all the way to your tailbone.

The middle layer is a muscular layer. This layer consists of longer, slightly thicker muscles which can span across two to five vertebrae. In the lower back, this middle layer also includes two abdominal muscles which 'swing around' from our abdomen and attach to the vertebrae of the lower back. These important abdominal muscles will be described in more detail shortly.

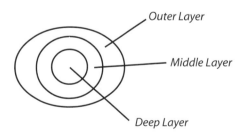

The outer layer, closest to the skin and furthest from the spine, is also a muscular layer. These are the big 'power' muscles which create the larger movements of the spine. They are thick and heavy and can span across ten or more vertebrae. These are the muscles strengthened by traditional back and abdominal exercises.

The Deep Layer

The deep layer consists of the vertebrae of the spine, the spinal discs and ligaments and a series of small muscles which run from one vertebrae to the next. The discs and ligaments perform two functions: helping to stabilize the spinal column and providing the brain with information about the exact position of every joint and vertebrae in the spine. The small, single level muscles found in the deep layer also generate this position or *postural* information.

The Middle Layer

Four key muscles of the middle layer provide the bulk of the stability required to keep our lower back working effectively and without pain. Two of these are back muscles and two are abdominal muscles. Their names are not important but some people do like to know these things. The stabilizing muscles which are found in the back are the *multifidus* and the *quadratus lumborum*. The stabilizers which come from the abdominal group are the *internal oblique* and the *transversus abdominis*.

The Outer Layer

This is the layer of large, thick and long muscles which are found just below the skin. These muscles can create large amounts of power and they come into play when we are straightening up from a bent position, moving from laying on our back to sitting up or when lifting very heavy objects. The outer layer muscles of the back are collectively known as the *erector spinae* muscles. Two further abdominal muscles, the *external oblique* and the *rectus abdominis*, are also components of this final layer.

Basic Function of the Spine

To this point the back has been described as being made up of three layers with each layer performing a specific task related to optimal function of the spine. Let's look at each of these in more detail especially in terms of how each is related to back injury and pain.

The Deep Layer

Our spinal column consists of 25 vertebrae held together by discs, ligaments and muscles. With every movement of our body the spine bends and rotates at the roughly seventy five joints found throughout the spinal column.

This is easily appreciated when we reach down to pick up a golf ball or when we reach into the back seat of our car to check the seat belt of our young son or daughter. Less obvious is the fact that some amount of bending and rotating occurs when we walk, sit or even raise our arm above our head.

These spinal motions come in two varieties - small and large. The larger bending and rotating motions are what we see if we look at an x-ray of a spine. With an x-ray we can see the relative position of individual vertebrae and the degree to which each is bending or rotating. The small motions are so small they are not observable even with an x-ray (although they have been measured in research laboratories using specialized equipment). The smaller spinal motions occur in the horizontal plane only and are sometimes referred to as 'slides'. They can be thought of as the building blocks of the larger bending and rotating motions of the spine.

For example, in order for the large motion of left side bending to occur between two vertebrae, a very small amount of right side 'slide' must also occur. On an x-ray we would see the larger left side bend, but not the tiny 'slide' to the right.

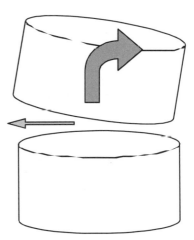

With regard to movement of the spine the function of the deep layer is twofold. First, the ligaments of the deep layer serve to limit the size or amplitude of the larger bending and rotating motions. In keeping with the door hinge analogy, the ligaments act like a door stop - they prevent the vertebrae from moving too far in any direction. If these large motions were not kept within certain limits effective and painfree spinal movement would not be possible.

Secondly, the discs, small muscles and ligaments of the deep layer have the ability to 'sense' changes in the position of the many joints of the spinal column and send this postural information to the brain. Scientists, physical therapists and doctors have long appreciated the importance of the stabilization provided by spinal ligaments. However, we are just now beginning to understand the significance of the position-sensing function of the deep layer. Indeed, it appears that our brain is extremely dependent on this postural information when attempting to effectively organize and use the various muscles which make our spine work.

To illustrate this idea, lets use a simple analogy. Imagine you are driving your car along a busy downtown street. Cars, pedestrians, traffic lights, and people on bicycles all vie for your attention. Your eyesight provides you with critical positional information about your car relative to the other people in the street. As you are driving, a blindfold is suddenly slipped over your eyes, preventing you from seeing all this activity. How confident would you feel in continuing to drive your car when you couldn't see what was going on around you? Most of us would immediately take our foot off the gas and apply the brakes until we could see again.

In order to drive a car safely, we require a constant stream of information about our position relative to other vehicles and to other people in the street. Likewise, our brain needs a steady stream of accurate information about the relative position of all our joints if it is going to successfully 'drive' the muscles of our body.

When deprived of this information, our brain often chooses to 'shut off' certain muscles just as we would take our foot off the gas if we were suddenly blindfolded while driving. Unfortunately, this 'shutting off' of muscles occurs following most types of spinal injury and can lead to further injury as our spinal joints, discs and nerves are left unsupported.

Spine Injury and the Deep Layer ...

Recent research has clearly shown that the spine's sliding, bending and rotating motions must be well controlled to avoid back injury. With damage to virtually any part of the spinal column these motions can become too large, and we feel this as back pain. Our body uses muscles to control the small sliding motions, but to control them, our brain needs to somehow 'know' that the motions are occurring in the first place.

In order to activate the correct muscles to control motion at a spinal joint, our brain must be 'aware' of the position and motion occurring at that joint, just as you need to be aware of the activity in the street before stepping on the gas pedal of your car. For this purpose, the spinal discs, ligaments and small muscles of the spine's *deep layer* contain tiny nerves which send this positional information to the brain. This constitutes part of what is commonly thought of as our 'sense of balance'.

Every split second, spinal discs, along with the ligaments and small muscles at every joint in the body send this positional information to the brain so our brain can know where the different parts of our body are relative to each other. With this information, the brain can then activate the correct muscles to either create a certain movement or prevent a joint from sliding, bending or rotating too far in one direction.

As mentioned above, new research has shown quite conclusively that when the small sliding, bending and rotating motions of the spine are not kept under precise control, injury will occur. The injury may involve the vertebrae itself, a ligament, or the spinal disc. Therefore, developing a highly tuned 'positional sense' through our spine is the first step to rehabilitating or preventing back injury. It is this aspect of stabilization training which is so unique; the majority of the exercises will, to some extent, require us to use our balance sense more so than standard exercises.

Previous exercise approaches for back pain and for sports conditioning have essentially ignored position sense training. As we will see in coming sections, exercises designed to improve our position sense can be progressed from easy to extremely difficult ensuring that everyone can benefit from this aspect of the program.

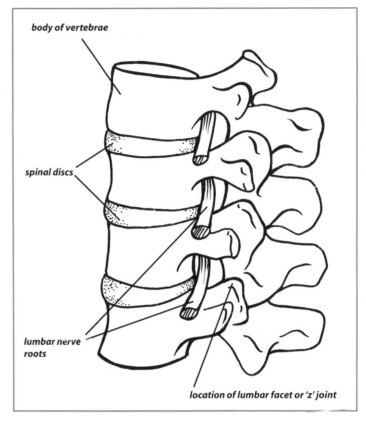

Four of the five lumbar vertebrae shown from the left side.

Like strength or aerobic fitness, balance is something we can improve with practice. The first part of the exercise program presented in this book will concentrate on improving our position sense through our spine. Once we have developed a better awareness of balance or position through our spine, we will move on to the second stage - training the stabilizing muscles.

The Middle Layer - Stabilizing the Spinal Column

The job of stabilizing the spinal column (that is, preventing excessive motion at individual spinal joints) is left to the spinal ligaments of the deep layer and the muscles of the middle layer. Until recently we failed to appreciate the importance of the *middle layer* muscles in this activity, thinking that the ligaments did all the work of stabilizing the spine.

We now know that the ligaments only provide stability at the extreme end range of a movement. It is the middle layer muscles which are responsible for the majority of the stabilization required to keep our back functioning properly.

To understand the role of the middle layer muscles, imagine a nine month old toddler attempting the relatively simple act of standing and lifting one arm above his head. Let's say that at this age he has just enough balance skill to stand for a few seconds without support. We can guess that as he tries to raise his arm above his head, he is likely to fall.

He falls because as his arm is lifted, his body's balance point - his center of mass - shifts slightly. This shift of his center of mass changes the load on his spinal column. As his joint position sensing and muscle control systems are not well coordinated yet, his body can't cope with this change and he tumbles.

Most adults of course take these simple movements for granted yet a complicated set of muscle activations must take place in order to maintain spinal stability while our body is in motion.

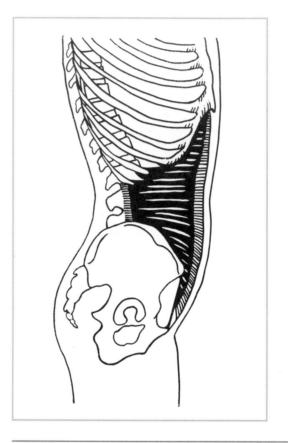

Transversus Abdominus - a middle layer stabilizing muscle, shown from the right side

When we are very young, our body learns to *pre-activate* the middle layer muscles before virtually any form of movement. This has the effect of bracing or stabilizing our spine so that movement in our limbs can occur efficiently and without disturbing our overall sense of balance. The degree to which the middle layer muscles are activated depends on the type of movement occurring in the body and the intensity of the movement. Larger, more forceful movements will require greater amounts of stabilization of the spine in order to minimize motion of the vertebrae.

Our trunk, or our *core*, as some therapists say, is the foundation of our entire body. The trunk acts like a platform from which our legs and arms function. If this platform is unstable, the arms and legs will have to work harder to accomplish a given task.

If we think of our trunk and right arm acting as a unit to lift something, we can imagine them as being similar to a crane on a construction site with its tall vertical tower and horizontal arm. If the base of our crane was built on soft sand we can appreciate how poorly it would work compared to another crane built on a concrete base. Even with a powerful motor to do the actual lifting, the entire structure might come crashing down if the base was unstable. Likewise, it doesn't matter how strong our shoulder, chest or outer layer muscles of our back might be if our trunk stabilizers are weak.

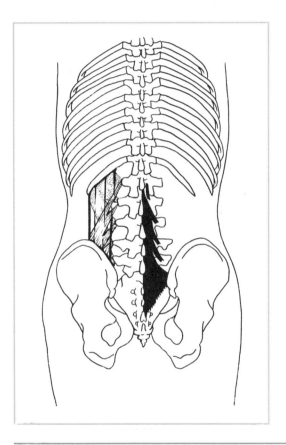

Middle layer stabilizing muscles: on the left, quadratus lumborum; on the right, multifidus

The trunk, functioning as the foundation on which our arms and legs operate, must be stable to allow our limbs to work at optimal efficiency. If our spine is not well stabilized, some part of the body will eventually become injured.

The fact that 80% of North Americans will one day experience a significant back injury suggests that we in the medical and rehabilitation professions have been going about this in the wrong way. Our focus on the large power muscles of the trunk has left many patients and athletes physically unprepared for their work or sport activities. As many of my physical therapy colleagues are already aware, even some of the shoulder, elbow, hip and knee problems our patients develop can be traced to poor stabilization of their spinal column.

The Software Crash Theory of Back Injury

Virtually everyone who works with computers has experienced the frustration of an operating system 'crash'. For some reason, the basic software program that runs the computer simply freezes or shuts down, resulting in a 'crashed system'. While some operating systems seem more 'crash-prone' than others, in fact no operating system is immune to this form of computer glitch and a crashed system will happen to most people once in a while. In 1997, a Canadian researcher named Stuart McGill conducted an experiment which, by accident, captured a similar phenomena - although in this case, the operating system was the central nervous system of one of his subjects.

Dr. McGill was studying the activation pattern of various trunk muscles during a series of weight lifting movements. He had a trained Olympic-style weightlifter in his laboratory and was recording the exact timing patterns with which the weightlifter's nervous system activated muscles throughout his trunk. After a few successful lifts, the weightlifter suddenly experienced a tremendous injury and could not continue. When the timing information was later reviewed, McGill noticed that at the precise time of the injury, a muscle which had been turned on during the previously successful lifts had failed to turn on for some reason. This meant that a single level of the weightlifter's spine was left unsupported for a moment leading to his injury. In this fleeting moment of sub-optimal stabilization, one of his lumbar vertebrae had over-rotated by a mere 0.5 degrees, resulting in an injury to a spinal ligament. His middle layer stabilizing muscles were not activated at the correct time and he had sustained a significant injury to his spine.

I refer to this as the *Software Crash Theory* of back injury. Just as a computer's operating system can occasionally and for no apparent reason fail to work correctly, Dr. McGill's unfortunate weightlifter demonstrated that the human 'operating system' may suffer the same sort of problem from time to time. This would seem to explain why so many patients tell us that the activity or movement which led to their injury was a movement or activity they had performed safely many times previously.

Once in a while, a complicated computer operating system is simply going to fail, and it may be that our spinal operating system will, from time to time, suffer similar glitches. If our computer's operating system was not well developed in the first place it will likely crash more frequently. Likewise, if we fail to develop or train the various components of our spinal operating system, we may also experience more frequent 'crashes'.

Fortunately, our spinal operating system is much more user friendly than is our computer's operating system. While we can only hit the restart button on our computer and await the next software crash, we can train and improve our spinal operating system through exercise. If we can 'fine tune' the spinal operating system through specialized exercise-based training, perhaps we can lessen our risk of the 'software crash' style of back injury. At the very least, we can likely recover more quickly from these and other types of back injury if our stabilizing muscles and position sensors are more finely tuned.

A Final Thought on the Middle Layer ...

When a back injury does occur, our normally logical body does something very irrational indeed. Researchers in Australia and Japan have shown that when a part of the spine is injured, a key stabilizing muscle (the *multifidus*) which would normally protect the injured joint, quickly shrinks. This has been shown to occur as rapidly as 24 hours following spinal injury. This means that just when the spine needs extra help, the muscles which would normally supply that help become smaller and weaker. This makes exercises designed to specifically strengthen these stabilizing muscles even more critical to a successful rehabilitation program.

The second and most important part of the exercise program described in this book will focus on improving the strength and function of the middle layer muscles. Chapters 6 and 7 will look at the role of the middle layer stabilization muscles in back injury prevention programs and conditioning programs for athletes.

The Outer Layer - Powering the Large Movements of the Spine

Once the spine has been stabilized by the middle layer muscles, the larger muscles of the back's outer layer can be trained for their role in lifting, bending and sports activities. Many 'old school' back strengthening exercises designed to rehabilitate or prevent back injury worked these muscles as opposed to the middle layer muscles. While the large outer layer muscles are certainly important, it is the middle layer muscles which are more involved in preventing back injury. Once again, Dr. McGill's Olympic weightlifter provides a good example of the important difference between the function and importance of the middle and outer spinal layers.

McGill's weightlifter would have had extremely strong outer layer muscles as these are the muscles used to lift these huge amounts of weight. It is unlikely however that he had sufficient middle layer stabilization of his spine. These were the muscles that 'crashed' and led to his injury.

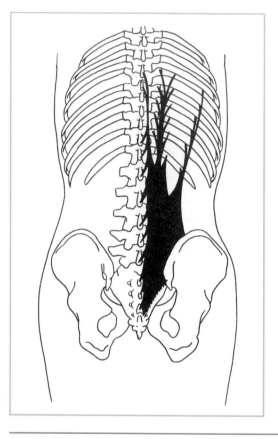

Erector Spinae: the primary outer layer muscle of the back. This muscle is found on both sides of the back and covers the middle layer muscles.

This then is the primary reason that old style back exercise programs often failed - we were spending all our time training muscles which moved the spine, but we neglected to train those muscles which stabilize and protect it.

Chapter 1 Key Points

1. ***Stabilization of the spinal joints is necessary for a healthy spine:***

   - our spinal column is inherently unstable - it is entirely dependent on specific muscles to maintain an upright posture and support our body weight during movement
   - the many small joints of the spine constantly move in sliding, bending and rotating directions - when these motions become too large, injury will occur to the vertebrae, discs or ligaments
   - the individual joints of the spinal column must be stabilized or stiffened in order for the overall spine to move efficiently and safely

2. ***Our 'trunk' can be thought of as being made up of three layers, each with a specific function:***

   - the deep layer consists of the vertebrae, the spinal discs and ligaments and the very small spinal muscles
   - the function of the deep layer is to provide *position sense* information to the brain regarding the position of the joints of the spinal column
   - the ligaments of the deep layer also stabilize the joints of the spinal column at extremes of movements such as bending and rotating
   - the middle layer of the trunk consists of medium size muscles responsible for stabilizing the joints of the spine in all postures
   - the outer layer is made up of large powerful muscles which can move the spine and create powerful motions of the trunk

3. ***Position sense is necessary for a healthy spine:***

   - our brain must know the exact position of every joint in the spine in order to correctly activate the stabilizing muscles of the spine
   - when we train our spine's joint position sense, we fine tune our brain's ability to detect and react to the small sliding, bending and rotating motions occurring throughout the spinal column
   - a more finely tuned movement detection sense allows our brain to use the correct stabilizing muscles more effectively, protecting our spinal column from injury

4. ***Our trunk or core is the platform or foundation from which all forms of physical activity begin:***

   - our arms and legs require a solid, stable base from which to operate
   - if our core is unstable, the shoulder and hip muscles often have to work excessively, potentially leading to tendonitis-type problems in these areas
   - even if the shoulder and hip muscles remain healthy, the back will often be injured if the core is unstable

5. **_Old style abdominal exercises such as sit-ups and most back strengthening exercises fail to train the stabilizing muscles:_**

- sit ups do not train the spine stabilizing abdominal muscles, especially the _transversus abdominis_ (TrA)
- old style back strengthening exercises emphasize the powerful outer layer of the back but do not train the more important middle layer (especially the _transversus abdominus_ and the _multifidus_)
- these exercises also fail to train the deep layer for its job of providing position sense information to the brain

Chapter 2
Understanding Your Back Pain ... What does my diagnosis mean?

Most people are unfamiliar with the medical terms used to describe both the part of their body which has been injured and the nature of the injury itself. The following is a brief outline of the terms used to identify the more common causes of low back pain. The relative benefits which may be reasonably expected of stabilization training in each diagnosis are also discussed.

Disc-Related Back Pain

Back pain caused by a bulging or herniated spinal disc is relatively rare. In fact only about 3 to 5% of people with low back pain have a bulging spinal disc. When this problem does occur, the disc puts pressure on a spinal nerve root resulting in the person's back and leg pain. In the case of true disc-related back pain, the disc between two vertebrae, for example the fourth and fifth lumbar vertebrae, develops a bulge which puts pressure on the large nerve passing just behind the disc.

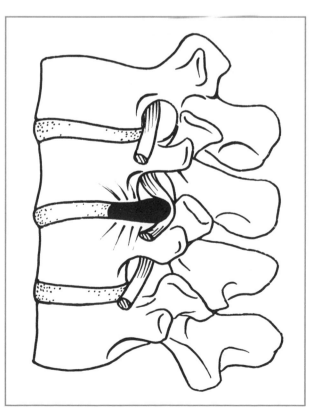

The lumbar spine shown from the left demonstrating a herniated disc between the third and fourth lumbar vertebrae

Usually (but not always) the person with actual disc-related back pain will have leg pain which is worse than their back pain along with numbness and muscle weakness somewhere in the lower leg or foot. These people will almost always have changes in their normal muscle reflexes as well.

Unfortunately, many people with less severe back problems are told they have a *slipped disc* or *sciatica*. For the record, spinal discs do not 'slip' out of place and 'sciatica' is a vague term which only describes back pain which spreads down the leg. Leg pain may or may not be due to an injured spinal disc and is therefore not diagnostic in and of itself for disc-related back pain.

Stabilization Training and Disc-Related Back Pain

This is one of the more serious types of back injury treated by physical therapists since it has the potential to require corrective surgery whereas most other back problems do not. That said, surgeons today seem more willing to try non-surgical approaches (i.e., physical therapy) before suggesting an operation. Whether a person's early management involves surgery or not, the goal of treatment is to alleviate the compression on the nerve root. In many instances this can be accomplished non-surgically; however, if the degree of disc injury is too severe (in the case, for instance, of a massive herniation of the disc), surgery will likely be neccessary.

Spinal stabilization exercises are not the primary, acute-stage form of treatment for true disc-related back pain. Stabilization exercises should not begin until compression of the spinal nerve has been completely relieved. Once the nerve root compression is resolved (either by surgery or physical therapy techniques) stabilization training will be very beneficial in terms of strengthening the middle layer muscles which provide the primary support and protection for the spine and the injured disc.

Researchers have shown that following disc injury, an important stabilizing muscle of the spine (the *multifidus*) quickly shrinks, becoming weak. Surprisingly, this has been shown to happen as early as twenty four hours following injury. This is an example of the 'shutting-down' phenomena described in the last chapter. Other researchers have noted that without specific training, these muscles do not recover their proper function even five years following the initial injury.

Stabilization exercises which target the middle layer are the best exercise option we have to offset these problems and ensure an optimal recovery from injury. Australian researchers have demonstrated that spinal stabilization exercises will re-train the multifidus and restore it to its pre-injury level of function much more quickly and completely than traditional methods.

Mechanical Back Pain

Mechanical low back pain has become a catch-all phrase for a number of different injuries involving the many joints, discs, ligaments and muscles of the spine. Physical therapists prefer to use terms which we feel more specifically describe the actual injury sustained by the patient. We use these terms based on our ability to use 'hands-on' manual therapy assessment methods to determine the extent to which the various joints and muscles of the spine are functioning correctly.

Sprain

The term *sprain* specifically describes an injury to a spinal ligament due to some form of fall, twist or other accident. A ligament does not become injured without trauma, as ligaments are strong structures which require a decent amount of force before they are stretched or torn. In that ligaments help stabilize the small bending and rotating motions of the spinal joints, an injured ligament may allow a joint to move too much in any one direction, resulting in pain.

Strain

Similar to a ligament sprain, a *strain* always occurs due to some kind of trauma but involves a muscle. Like ligaments, healthy muscles do not tear unless subjected to a significant force. It is not possible to wake up one morning with a true muscle strain if you cannot recall some kind of accident. Usually, the person with a true muscle strain injury will have experienced some kind of traumatic event and have felt pain immediately. Sprains and strains will vary in degree or severity based on the extent to which the ligament or muscle fibres are torn.

Subluxation

This refers to a joint injury where a small spinal joint becomes 'stuck' in a certain position and is unable to move fully through its bending and rotating motions. Subluxation may occur with or without trauma. The injury sustained by Dr. McGill's weightlifter (see page 13) is an example of a subluxation injury. The weightlifter's spinal joint moved only 0.5 degrees upon injury. This is not enough excess or abnormal movement to be noticed on a spinal x-ray but it clearly demonstrates that a very small amount of incorrect spinal motion can lead to significant injury and pain. Subluxations may occur at any level of the spine, including the large sacroiliac joints that join the base of the spine (the *sacrum*) to the right and left halves of the pelvis.

Hypermobility

This term also refers to a joint problem; however, unlike subluxations where the joint becomes 'stuck', the hypermobile joint develops *too much* motion. Usually the hypermobile spinal joint has, for some reason, lost the normal degree of stabilization provided by its ligaments. This leads to greater than normal amounts of bending and rotating at the joint. Hypermobilities may be due to injury, certain forms of athletic training (e.g., gymnastics) or the fact that some people are just born with 'loose joints'. A hypermobile joint may remain relatively painless if the stabilizing muscles protecting the joint are able to control the excessive amount of motion.

Instability

A joint which has become unstable no longer has adequate stabilization from either its ligaments or its stabilizing muscle. Therefore the hypermobile joint described above can become an unstable joint if the stabilizing muscles acting at the joint lose their ability to adequately limit or control the amount of movement at the joint. Unstable joints tend to be very painful and are generally made worse with movement, although the type of movement which creates pain may be quite inconsistent.

Osteoarthritis

Osteoarthritis (OA) is a wear and tear problem involving the protective layer of cartilage which lines our joints. Everyone will have developed some degree of osteoarthritis by the age of sixty, simply because our joints wear out somewhat over time. As cartilage does not contain any pain nerves, healthy joint cartilage can tolerate significant compression forces without the joint becoming painful. Unfortunately, this protective layer wears thin over time leaving the bone underneath the cartilage exposed to the compression forces which occur normally with all movement.

Since bone does have pain nerves, these compression forces can lead to significant amounts of pain. Joints which seem to become most painful with OA are the large joints such as the hip and knee. These joints need to tolerate compression forces in the range of *eight to ten times* our body weight during activities like running or walking up a flight of stairs.

Osteoarthritic changes are also quite common in the joints of the lower back and neck. This creates two problems from a spinal stability perspective; the increased pain and the loss of smoothness of the joint surfaces. Both the pain and the roughening of the joint surfaces lead to weakness of the stabilizing muscles which normally act at the arthritic joint. This usually results in even greater amounts of pain and thus even weaker muscles. Gentle stabilization and stretching exercises are the best exercise prescription for people with more severe OA-related problems. A physical therapist will be an excellent resource in choosing the safest, most effective exercises to control this type of back pain.

Stabilization Training and Mechanical Back Pain

Sprains, strains, subluxations and osteoarthritic problems may require other forms of treatment in the initial stages to safely and effectively resolve the problem. A physical therapist can discuss the most suitable options for each person's injury. Once the initial injury has begun to heal, stabilization exercises may be added to the treatment program. Each person's home exercise program should consist of various stabilization exercises designed as specifically as possible for their condition and their activities.

Today, hypermobilities and instabilities are treated primarily with stabilization training. The obstacle here is the fact that as the joint becomes unstable the 'deep layer' of the spine has a more difficult time sending accurate positional information to the brain. Without good quality positional information it becomes harder for the brain to activate the very stabilizing muscles required to solve the problem. For this reason especially, hypermobilities and instabilities are very difficult to manage. A great commitment on the part of the patient is required in order to keep their problem under control.

It is essential that people with spinal instability perform their stabilization exercises faithfully. If they do not, their pain will return. In some extreme cases, the instability is too severe to correct with exercise, and surgery may be required. In these cases, once the person has recovered sufficiently from their surgery, they should begin stabilization exercises under the guidance of a licensed physical therapist.

Degenerative Disc Disease

Our spinal discs have a variety of functions, one of which is to act as a cushion or shock absorber for the spinal column. As we get older, the discs lose some of their elasticity and become more brittle. At the same time discs lose some of their height. There is disagreement in the medical profession as to where the pain of degenerative disc disease comes from. Some feel the thinner disc leads to greater stress on the facet joints of the vertebrae (see diagram, page 8) resulting in a painful arthritis of these joints. Others feel the more brittle disc itself becomes the source of pain as tiny cracks develop within the structure of the disc.

Stabilization Training and Degenerative Disc Disease

As with spinal osteoarthritis, degenerative disc disease cannot be 'cured' by either medical or rehabilitative means; however, the pain associated with these conditions can be reduced, sometimes quite significantly, by re-training the muscles to do their proper job. If the stabilizing muscles can be made effective again, the abnormal motions of the small spinal joints can be brought under control, resulting in decreased pain.

Spondylolithesis (spaun-di-lo-lie-thee-sis)

The vertebrae of the spine can be thought of as having a front and rear half. The front half consists of a large cylindrical part called the *body*. The rear half is made up of the 'tube' which surrounds the spinal cord along with three odd-looking projections to which muscles and ligaments attach. In a very small number of people, the portion of the vertebrae where the front and back halves meet develops incorrectly. In these unusual vertebrae, the region where the front and back halves attach is actually formed of a thick, heavy connective tissue instead of bone. Sometimes these areas of connective tissue can let go, allowing the front half of the vertebrae to separate slightly from the back half.

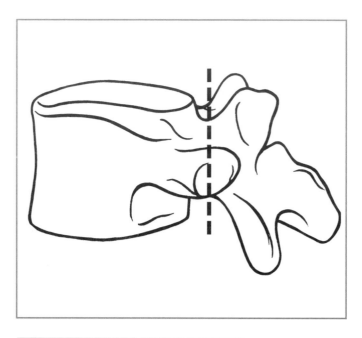

In spondylolithesis the front half of the vertebrae separates from the rear half along this line

Stabilization Training and Spondylolithesis

For people with this condition, spinal stabilization exercises can provide some of the best pain control available. As with instabilities and OA, spondylolithesis provides a great challenge to the position sensors (deep layer) of the spine. Thus, while stabilization training can be effective, it must be performed regularly in order to be helpful in this situation.

Spinal Stenosis

If we were to look down the length of the spinal column from above, we would see that the shape of the individual vertebrae allows for the spinal column to have a hollow centre, like a paper towel tube. In reality, the 'hollow' centre is where the spinal cord is found. Therefore the spinal cord, carrying all the messages between our brain and body, is located inside a circular 'tube' of bone formed by the vertebrae.

In a small percentage of older people, this tube begins to get more narrow as new, abnormal bone growth occurs inside the *spinal canal* where the spinal cord is located. This can lead to a variety of problems from pain to numbness to muscular weakness.

Stabilization Training and Spinal Stenosis

Unfortunately, there is very little that can be done to correct the actual problem of spinal stenosis. The narrowing of the spinal canal will not be affected by any form of exercise nor any form of medical treatment presently available. Stabilization training may help people with this condition to function better and they may have some improvement in their symptoms with stronger stabilization muscles.

This is a complicated medical condition and thus any rehabilitative exercise program should be designed by a licensed physical therapist familiar with stabilization training.

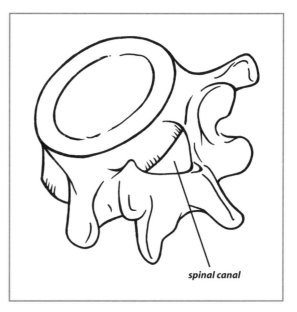

spinal canal

The spinal canal becomes more narrow in spinal stenosis

Rheumatoid Arthritis (RA)

Rheumatoid or Inflammatory Arthritis is a serious medical problem which can affect almost any system of the body. The joints, lungs, kidneys, eyes and hearts of people with RA may develop various problems related to this disease. While not completely understood, RA is currently thought to be a form of autoimmune disease. This means that the body apparently fails to recognize its own tissues and initiates a self-destructive process. Because of the wide range of possible complications, this condition should be managed by a medical specialist trained specifically in RA-related conditions.

From the joint perspective, the disease process can effect virtually any joint in the body. RA damages and eventually destroys the tissues found within the joints, namely the protective cartilage and some of the ligaments. This type of damage leaves the joint very unstable, and therefore quite vulnerable and in need of protection. For this and other reasons it is important that people who have been diagnosed with RA be treated by a medical rheumatologist, and when necessary, a physical therapist.

Low Back Pain, Stabilization Training and Rheumatoid Arthritis

An interesting feature of RA is the fact that it almost never causes low back pain. Dr. Evelyn Sutton, a Halifax rheumatologist stated "while I try never to say never with regard to anything medical, rheumatoid arthritis should never be blamed as the cause of someone's back pain. This isn't to say that a person with RA can't have low back pain, it simply means their low back pain will be caused by something other than RA." Thus the person who has RA and low back pain needs to be examined by a health care professional to determine the reason for their sore back.

While stabilization therapy will often prove helpful for people with RA, each and every person with RA will experience a unique set of challenges related to their disease. For this reason it is best that the person with RA have a spinal stabilization program designed specifically for them. If you have been diagnosed with any form of rheumatoid arthritis, please consult with a licensed health care professional before beginning any exercise program.

Chapter 3
Essential Spinal Stabilization Concepts

Ideally, each person's spinal stabilization program should be a unique exercise *prescription* since the physical activity demands and injury history of each person will be unique. Although providing the same generic stabilization program for all people with a previous lumbar disc injury may at first seem reasonable, this approach simply doesn't lead to success as readily as does a more 'person specific' program.

For example, let's say that a 36 year-old airline pilot who was once a competitive figure skater and a 58 year-old accounts manager with no athletic background have each recovered from a spinal disc injury. The pilot now competes in triathalons while the accounts manager prefers walking for exercise. They will obviously have different physical demands placed on their spinal column and therefore, their stabilization programs need to be more tailored.

Instead of presenting a 'rehabilitation cookbook' with a collection of recipes to be followed by everyone, I will outline several important *concepts* which should be considered when designing a spinal stabilization program. People with back pain should consult with a physical therapist to design the safest and most effective program based on their type of injury, stage of recovery and their current physical ability. If you have a generally healthy, non-painful back, you may wish to put together your own program based on these concepts or you may wish to consult with a licensed physical therapist familiar with stabilization training.

To begin, we'll define some of the terms used throughout the next few sections.

Spinal Stabilization Definitions

Deep Layer Exercises

Exercises which develop position sense through our spine and extremities. These usually challenge our ability to maintain our balance in some way.

Middle Layer Exercises

Exercises which train the key stabilization muscles of the trunk. The stabilizing abdominals are the internal oblique and transversus abdominis. The stabilizing back muscles are the multifidus and quadratus lumborum. The middle layer exercises are further divided into two groups - *static and dynamic*.

Static middle layer stabilization exercises are exercises which require us to hold a certain position or posture without movement. *Dynamic* middle layer stabilization exercises are exercises which require us to create movement somewhere in our body while maintaining a stable trunk or core.

Outer Layer Exercises

Exercises which develop the power muscles of the trunk. People who play very physical sports such as hockey, football and rugby or who have very physically demanding jobs (e.g., forestry workers) may need to spend more time on these exercises than people with more sedentary lives or whose sports are not quite as hard on the body.

Base of Support

The distance between two or more parts of your body which are in contact with a supporting surface such as the floor. For example, when you stand with your feet spread shoulder width apart, you have a wider base of support than when you stand with your feet together. Standing on only one foot reduces your base of support to the area under your foot. A wider base of support is a more stable base of support; a more narrow base of support is a less stable base of support.

Points of Stable Contact

The number of connections we have through our body to a stable surface. For example, standing with two feet on the ground provides two stable points of contact. Standing on one foot provides only one stable point of contact while kneeling on a large ball provides no stable point of contact. Kneeling on a large ball while holding on to a wall with one hand provides a single point of stable contact.

Essential Trunk Stabilization Concepts

Concept 1:
Stabilization exercises and general daily activities should not exceed a person's stabilization ability.

Researchers have determined that spinal injury occurs when the muscles of the spine are no longer able to stabilize the joints of the spinal column; therefore, it is imperative that people perform exercises which do not overwhelm the capabilities of their stabilizing muscles. This is true of both stabilization exercises and other daily activities. For example, a person with a moderate degree of stabilizing ability may be able to tolerate a brisk walk for aerobic exercise but they may not be able to stabilize their spine while jogging. Likewise, a injured worker may be sufficiently stable to perform a lifting activity involving 10 kg loads but not 15 kg loads.

When we perform exercises or physical activities which overwhelm our stabilization ability, the body will attempt to use the outer layer muscles as stabilizers. Because these large movement muscles are not designed for stabilization functions, this often leads to further mechanical problems and possibly increased pain. This represents a faulty movement pattern and should be avoided whenever possible. This brings us to concept 2.

Concept 2:
Quality of movement before quantity of movement.

The overall goal of stabilization training is to teach our body to make correct use of the deep, middle and outer layer muscles. To achieve this goal, we must perform the exercises with an emphasis on technique rather than a high number of repetitions. Similarly, exercises which are too difficult for us (see Concept 1) will create too significant a challenge for our stabilization muscles and will cause our body to compensate by using outer layer muscles in an attempt to meet the stability demands of the exercise.

As tempting as it may be to progress through the exercise levels quickly, please be sure that you are completely capable of performing each exercise correctly before moving to more challenging variations.

Essential Trunk Stabilization Concepts ...

Concept 3:

Start with simple exercises and gradually add more challenging exercises as your technique permits.

Begin by performing exercises emphasizing position sense and static stability (the deep and middle layer exercises) separately. When you become good at each of these, move onto exercises which combine position sense and static stability challenges in a single exercise. This involves holding a posture while on a SwissBall or wobble board. Finally, combine position sense and dynamic stability exercises for the greatest degree of stabilization challenge.

Concept 4:

Position sense or deep layer exercises are progressed (i.e., made more challenging) by decreasing the base of support and the number of points of stable contact.

As defined earlier, the base of support refers to the distance between your feet or hands on the floor during exercises. The same exercise performed with a wide base of support will be more difficult if performed with a more narrow base of support. Likewise, the number of points of stable contact refers to the total number of hands or feet you have in contact with a stable surface (usually the floor) during any exercise. An exercise performed easily with three points of stable contact will be more difficult when attempted with only a single point of stable contact.

Position sense (deep layer) exercises may also be progressed by taking away our vision or by adding movement to the exercise. Most people are quite dependent on their vision to help maintain their balance; therefore, we can make the deep layer exercises much more difficult by performing the exercise with our eyes closed. In fact, any exercise performed with the eyes closed allows us to be more aware of our body and how it is moving or working.

Of course, exercising with the eyes closed should only be attempted if there is no risk of injury should you lose your ability to maintain the position. For example, many athletes are able to kneel on a large inflatable ball as a form of advanced deep layer training. If the person closes their eyes they will make the exercise much more difficult, but they will also be at higher risk of falling off the ball.

Deep layer position sense exercises may also be progressed by attempting to maintain our balance while moving our arms or legs.

Essential Trunk Stabilization Concepts ...

Concept 5 - Part 1:

Static stability exercises are progressed by holding each posture for longer periods of time while performing fewer repetitions

A static stabilization exercise is an exercise where we attempt to maintain a certain position or posture to train the endurance aspect of the spinal stabilizers. At first we might perform ten repetitions of the exercise, holding the position each time for five to ten seconds. To progress these, we would hold each position for longer periods of time, up to 30 or 45 seconds. As the length of time spent holding each position increases, the number of repetitions may decrease. Therefore we may begin doing a certain static stabilization exercise 10 times, holding each posture for 10 seconds. As the endurance of these muscles improves we might perform only three or four repetitions, but we would be holding each posture for up to 45 seconds.

A good measure of how long to hold each posture involves movement quality; hold each position for as long as you can maintain near-perfect technique. If you begin to lose optimal technique after ten seconds, perform a higher number of repetitions, stopping each when your technique begins to fail. As your endurance improves, you will find yourself holding positions for longer periods of time. As this happens, perform fewer repetitions.

Concept 5 - Part 2:

Dynamic stability exercises are progressed by performing more repetitions

Dynamic stabilization exercises require us to move in some way while maintaining a stable trunk or core. These exercises are progressed by performing more repetitions. Again, the key consideration is technique. Perform as many repetitions of a given dynamic stabilization exercise as you can until your technique begins to fail. When you have done several repetitions and can no longer do the exercise with perfect form, stop. If you find yourself performing more than twenty repetitions of a given dynamic stabilization exercise with excellent technique, it may be time to move on to a more challenging exercise.

Concept 6

Avoid any exercise which increases your back or neck pain.

In chapter 1 we discussed the fact that following spinal joint injury, the body often responds by 'shutting down' the stabilization muscles near the site of the injury. This occurs via two similar but distinct mechanisms.

Essential Trunk Stabilization Concepts ...

Concept 6 (continued)

Researchers have shown that when swelling (fluid) builds up within a joint, the stabilizing muscle of that joint stops working. For example, at a large joint like the knee, the quadriceps muscle will start to have difficulty contracting with as little as one tablespoon (15 - 20 ml) of fluid within the joint. With almost any form of acute joint injury, including spinal injury, there will be some amount of swelling within the joint. Unfortunately, where there is joint swelling, there is muscle deactivation, usually affecting the middle layer muscles at the injured joint.

The other mechanism which appears to lead to this deactivation of stabilizing muscle involves pain. Less is known about the process by which pain causes a shut-down of stabilizing muscle; however, it is a common problem, especially in the acute stage of an injury.

While we see a shutting-down of the nearby middle layer muscle with many acute joint injuries, we often see an increase in the activity of the outer layer muscles which move the injured joint. This is commonly described as muscle spasm. Muscle spasm is often thought to be the primary problem when it is observed in someone with an acute back injury. In fact, the muscle spasm is usually secondary to some other underlying injury, often involving a joint. For this reason, treatment aimed at resolving the spasm rarely solves the problem in that the spasm isn't really the problem; it is merely a complication of the underlying joint injury.

Since pain will often deactivate the stabilizing, middle layer muscles we wish to re-train, it is important not to push our exercises to the point of pain, especially in the early stages of recovery. There are many variations of these deep, middle and outer layer exercises. As such there should be no need to perform stabilization exercises which increase a person's pain. If a given exercise makes the pain worse, modify the exercise or perform some other exercise in its place which serves a similar purpose (i.e., position sense, stabilization or powerful movement). If this doesn't help, seek advice from a physical therapist.

Concept 7
Ideally, all stabilization exercises should be performed while maintaining a contraction of the transversus abdominis muscle.

A large amount of anatomical, biomechanical and postural control research has identified one specific abdominal muscle which seems to play a very important role in low back stabilization. The transversus abdominis (TrA) is the deepest of the four abdominal muscles and attaches directly to the spinal column.

Essential Trunk Stabilization Concepts ...

Concept 7 (continued)

If you were to imagine a corset or girdle wrapping around your waist, you would have an idea of how this muscle is built. Due to its direct spinal attachments, the TrA is able to stabilize individual vertebrae of the lower back, preventing the excess sliding, bending and rotating motions described earlier.

With its unique design and direct attachments to the spinal column, many physical therapists feel the TrA is the key to lumbar stabilization. Further studies have found that when we move an arm or leg (as when we are walking, reaching, kicking, etc.) the TrA 'turns on' *before* the actual arm or leg muscles which produce the limb movement. The TrA is both designed and used by the body to stabilize the lower spine so that movement of the arms and legs can occur more efficiently and with less stress on the spine itself.

The next chapter will describe the technique used to activate and train the TrA. While most people will be able to learn this technique, especially with the help of a licensed physical therapist, there will be some people who will struggle to 'activate' and strengthen this muscle. I would recommend that, despite the evidence regarding the importance of TrA, if you really cannot learn to activate this muscle, go on to the other deep, middle and outer layer exercises and follow the instructions provided by your physical therapist. I personally have treated several people who could not learn to contract their TrA, yet they went on to do very well using the remainder of the stabilization exercises.

Concept 8
Have fun with your exercise program!

When was the last time you met someone who just couldn't wait to do their traditional abdominal exercises? Even the most enthusiastic exercise nut still dreads the thought of doing endless sit-ups, crunches and oblique twists. Many more people have given up altogether because they find their neck or lower back hurts when they do these old-style exercises. The fact that an up-to-date spinal stabilization program is based on better and more reliable science is reason enough to try it. That people actually *enjoy* this approach is certainly unique when it comes to abdominal exercises.

The fact that spinal stabilization training often seems more like play than exercise means that people are much more likely to stay with it indefinitely. As people move into the moderate level exercises and begin using the large, inflatable 'swissballs', the little kid in each of us quickly recognizes the fun side to stabilization training.

Chapter 4
The Complete Spinal Stabilization Exercise Program

We've covered all the anatomy and science that relates to stabilization training. We know why it will help people control their back pain and how it will lead to improved athletic performance. But how do we actually do it? How do we learn to isolate and contract the transversus abdominis muscle and then use that contraction with all the other stabilization exercises?

Initial Stabilization using Transversus Abdominis

The transversus abdominis muscle is 'connected' via our nervous system to our 'pelvic floor muscles'. Because of this neurologic connection between the pelvic floor muscles and transversus abdominis, we can contract our pelvic floor muscles and automatically get some amount of contraction in the transversus abdominis. While we normally don't think too much about our 'pelvic floor', these are the muscles that we use to keep almost every form of liquid, gas and solid from escaping our body's lower regions.

To teach yourself to control your transversus abdominis lie on your back with your knees bent and your feet on the floor. Gently, then with gradually increasing effort, tighten your pelvic floor muscles as if you were trying to stop yourself from peeing (imagine a long line at the movie theatre washroom after *Schindler's List* and a pair of extra-large diet cokes). Most women who have had babies will recognize this as the *Kegel* exercise. Once you can do this consistently and without too much effort, the next step is to maintain this pelvic floor contraction and add the transversus abdominis.

To do this, visualize the transversus abdominis in its relaxed state as the top of a tent. As transversus abdominis contracts, the peak of the tent is drawn down and the tent spreads apart. Think of drawing your belly button down into your body, or pulling your abdomen away from the inside of your pants waistband.

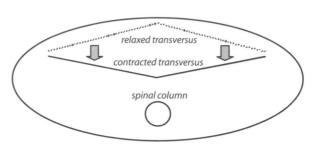

Therefore, isolating and contracting the transversus abdominis is a two part process. First, tighten your pelvic floor muscles; then, while maintaining that contraction, draw your lower abdomen inward, creating a bowl-shaped or concave lower belly.

One final thing: You must be able to do this while still breathing in a relaxed manner. Holding your breath while trying to exercise is generally not a good idea. The transversus abdominis and pelvic floor muscles must contract while you breathe gently and regularly. If this is the most difficult part of the process for you, don't worry - you are not alone. Most people take at least a few days to get this straightened out.

As mentioned in the last chapter, learning to properly contract transversus abdominis is probably the most difficult part of the entire stabilization program. It will usually help to have a physical therapist who is familiar with stabilization training coach you through this part of the process. A physical therapist can offer valuable and time-saving feedback on this and other parts of your stabilization program.

Once you can successfully isolate and contract your transversus abdominis, you are ready to begin your trunk stabilization program. Independent control of the transversus abdominis is probably important enough that each person should spend at least two weeks trying to learn the technique. If in that period you haven't quite mastered it, visit a local physical therapist who can help you. If after two or three weeks with the physical therapist you still haven't got it, I would suggest you move on to the remainder of the stabilization program. Perform the deep, middle and outer layer exercises as suggested by your physical therapist and maintain a 'neutral' low back posture during all exercises.

If you have had trouble learning to isolate the transversus abdominis and decide to begin exercises such as the entry-level deep and middle layer exercises, keep trying the transversus exercise. You never know when things will kick in.

Will this approach really work?

There are literally dozens of books and exercise methods available for the person with back pain which promise relief. The difference between these and the approach described in this book is that spinal stabilization is based on good science.

In the world of medical research, the most powerful form of scientific study is known as a multi-center trial. This involves not a single research team but a collection of independent research groups all looking at the same question. The major benefit of the multi-center trial is that it dramatically reduces the possibility of researcher error or bias.

The unique feature of spinal stabilization is that its basic foundations have been developed by a variety of researchers from around the world who were working *independently* of each other. Despite the lack of direct communication between these research teams, they have come to remarkably similar conclusions about the workings of the spine. These basic foundations have been described previously in this book but I will list them again for the sake of clarity:

1. *The spinal column - without muscle - is inherently unstable.*

2. *Spinal injury and a further decrease in spinal stability go hand in hand; it appears that one cannot occur without the other.*

3. *Specific muscles such as transversus abdominus, quadratus lumborum and multifidus provide the spine with the stability required for us to move safely and effectively. These muscles must activate at the correct time and to the correct degree to protect the spine from injury.*

4. *The multifidus muscle stops working once the spinal column is injured and does not recover fully even after the person's pain has improved.*

The key question then is, can the spinal stabilization exercise method described in this book actually reverse this problem and if so, will this lead to a healthier, less painful back? Research conducted in Australia suggests that indeed this approach does improve the function of the multifidus muscle and leads to a dramatic reduction in future episodes of back pain.

In 1996 Australian physiotherapists Julie Hides, Carolyn Richardson and Gwen Jull studied 39 people who had a sudden episode of low back pain. They divided these people into two groups; one group would be treated using a traditional approach and the other with the spinal stabilization approach designed by the physiotherapists. Over the first four weeks, both groups improved in terms of their pain and disability levels. The traditional treatment group did not see any improvement in the size or function of their multifidus muscle; 80% of the people in this group went on to have further episodes of back pain during the next year.

The people who performed the spinal stabilization exercises improved the size and function of their multifidus muscle in less than 6 - 8 weeks and only 30% of these people had recurrences of their back pain over the remainder of the year.

In 1997, another research team in Australia (O'Sullivan, Twomey, Allison) studied the effectiveness of spinal stabilization exercises with a group of 44 people with chronic back pain. Again the people were divided into spinal stabilization and traditional treatment groups. The people in the traditional treatment group did not see any improvement in their pain level or ability to perform everyday activities. The spinal stabilization group however saw a significant improvement in both their pain levels and functional abilities. This was maintained for over two years during the length of the study.

Will Spinal Stabilization Work for Me?

The research upon which the spinal stabilization approach is based and the studies which have been conducted to assess the effectiveness of this approach all suggest that spinal stabilization exercises will provide most people with the best opportunity to control their back pain and improve their ability to do what they want to do at work and in sports. Spinal stabilization exercises can therefore be expected to be a significant benefit to most people with low back pain.

Will there be some people who do not see a dramatic improvement in their symptoms? Unfortunately, the realistic answer must be yes; the reality of all forms of medical treatment is that no single approach is 100% effective for all people in all situations. Having accepted this reality, spinal stabilization remains the most advanced and sophisticated approach yet developed to control low back pain and improve spinal performance.

Spinal Stabilization and the Pelvic Tilt

For many years a variety of low back exercises and lifting techniques were taught which emphasized the 'pelvic tilt' posture. The pelvic tilt was thought to be a good posture to work from in that it supposedly activated the 'lower abdominals'. More recent research has shown that the pelvic tilt does not activate the transversus, internal oblique, quadratus lumborum or multifidus muscles. Further, the pelvic tilt posture actually *de*-stabilizes the spinal column by a small amount.

For these reasons, the pelvic tilt is no longer considered an effective position to work from for most people. The one group of back pain patients for whom the pelvic tilt may still be useful are those people with *spondylolithesis* (see page 19). For this select group, the pelvic tilt may still help with pain control.

Spinal Stabilization - The Exercises

Your physical therapist will help you correctly plan your exercise program based on your injury type, stage of recovery and stabilization ability. One or two exercises from each category (deep layer, middle layer and outer layer) should be included in your program. At all times, follow the instructions of your physical therapist and the basic concepts discussed in chapter 3.

At all times, choose exercises which challenge your current stabilization abilities without *overwhelming* your current stabilization abilities. An exercise is too advanced for your present stabilization potential if it causes pain or if you are unable to hold the posture for at least five seconds using excellent technique.

Once you have progressed to the exercises which make use of the SwissBall, you must remember to use a certain amount of caution and common sense. Exercises of any kind which are performed using these very unstable pieces of exercise equipment have the potential to cause serious injury if you fall or lose your balance. Perform your SwissBall exercises in an open area away from objects which could cause injury if you were to fall off the ball. Work with a reliable spotter when performing exercises which create a significant challenge to your balance or which could conceivably cause injury if you were to lose your balance.

Lastly, use a burst-resistant ball, especially if you are lifting weights while on the ball, to minimize your risk of serious injury should the ball be punctured. Burst-resistant balls are not puncture proof, but they are designed to deflate slowly should a hole develop in the ball.

Note:
The small open boxes beside each picture are intended to help therapists indicate to their patients which exercises are to be performed at a given point in their rehabilitation. Simply place a checkmark or 'X' in the box corresponding to the intended exercise. Using pencil is a good idea as the exercises used will likely change over time.

Deep Layer / Position Sense Exercises

These progress from easier to harder, therefore Deep Layer exercise 7 is more challenging than is Deep Layer exercise number 3. Concentrate on maintaining a quality TrA contraction throughout and try to hold each posture a few seconds longer every day.

1   **Single Leg Standing**

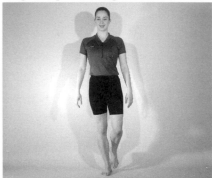

- with / without additional point of stable contact
- start by holding for a few seconds then build to 30 seconds
- when you can easily hold this position for 20 seconds, begin trying exercise 2, below

2   **Single Leg Standing**

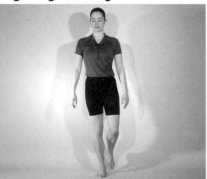

- eyes closed
- as with exercise 1, begin with a few seconds and gradually build to 30 seconds
- when you can easily hold this position for 20 seconds, begin trying exercise 3, below

3   **Single Leg Standing**

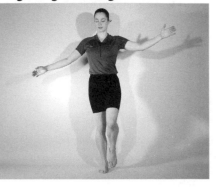

- eyes closed with arm movements
- begin with slow easy, symmetrical arm movements
- progress by moving the arms in different directions and at various speeds

Deep Layer / Position Sense Exercises

Progressing from easier to harder ... concentrate on maintaining a quality TrA contraction throughout and try to hold each posture a few seconds longer every day.

4   **Ball Sitting**

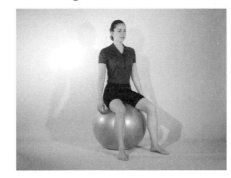

- eyes open, wide base of support
- practice maintaining balance while holding a transversus contraction
- try to sit for up to 5 minutes while holding a transversus contraction for up to 30 seconds then resting for 30 seconds

5   **Ball Sitting**

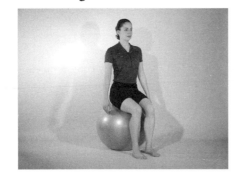

- eyes open, narrow base of support
- hold a transversus contraction
- try to sit for up to 5 minutes while holding a transversus contraction for up to 30 seconds then resting for 30 seconds

6   **Ball Sitting**

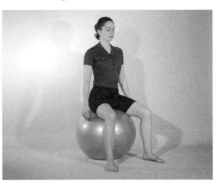

- eyes closed, wide base of support
- contract and hold as in exercises 4 and 5

40

Deep Layer / Position Sense Exercises

Progressing from easier to harder ... concentrate on maintaining a quality TrA contraction throughout and try to hold each posture a few seconds longer every day.

7   Ball Sitting

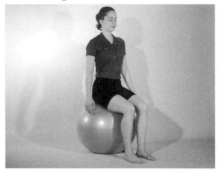

- eyes closed, narrow base of support
- contract TrA and hold as in exercises 4 and 5

8   Ball Sitting

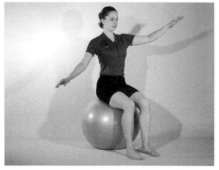

- eyes open, narrow base of support with arm movements
- contract TrA and hold

9   Ball Sitting

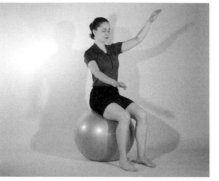

- eyes closed, narrow base of support with arm movements
- contract TrA and hold

Deep Layer / Position Sense Exercises

Progressing from easier to harder ... concentrate on maintaining a quality TrA contraction throughout and try to hold each posture a few seconds longer every day.

10 **Ball Sitting**

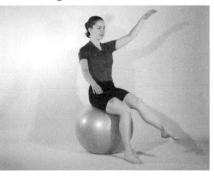

• eyes open, one point of stable contact
• contract and hold TrA

11 **Ball Sitting**

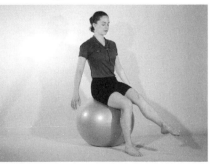

• eyes open, one point of stable contact, with arm movements
• contract and hold TrA

12 **Ball Sitting**

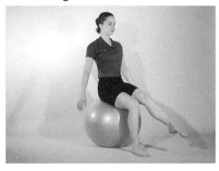

• eyes closed, one point of stable contact
• contract and hold TrA

Deep Layer / Position Sense Exercises
Progressing from easier to harder ... concentrate on maintaining a quality TrA contraction throughout and try to hold each posture a few seconds longer every day.

13   Ball Sitting

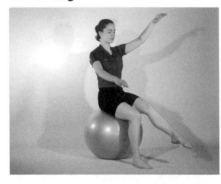

- eyes closed, one point of stable contact, with arm movements
- contract and hold TrA

14   Ball Sitting

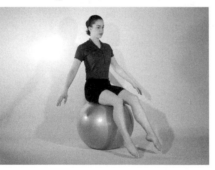

- no point of stable contact
- contract and hold TrA

15   Ball Sitting

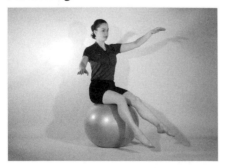

- no point of stable contact, add arm movements
- contract and hold TrA

Deep Layer / Position Sense Exercises

Progressing from easier to harder ... concentrate on maintaining a quality TrA contraction throughout and try to hold each posture a few seconds longer every day.

16   Ball Sitting

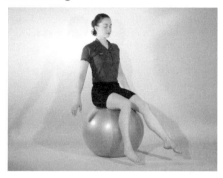

- no point of stable contact, eyes closed
- contract and hold TrA

17   Ball Sitting

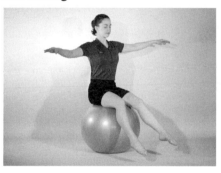

- no point of stable contact, eyes closed, add arm movements
- contract and hold TrA

18   Ball Kneeling

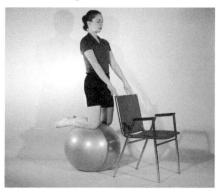

- two points of stable contact, eyes open
- contract and hold TrA

Hint:
To get up into a kneeling position on the ball, stand with the ball in front of you, resting between your knees. Your arms are reaching forward with your finger tips just touching the edge of the chair back. From this position, slowly roll up onto the ball, holding onto the chair back as soon as you begin to roll forward. As always, make sure someone is close by acting as a 'spotter'. Remember - do not use a chair which is on wheels as your 'stable' point of contact!

Deep Layer / Position Sense Exercises

Progressing from easier to harder ... concentrate on maintaining a quality TrA contraction throughout and try to hold each posture a few seconds longer every day.

19   **Ball Kneeling**

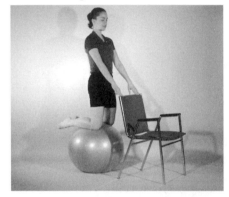

- two points of stable contact, eyes closed
- contract and hold TrA

20   **Ball Kneeling**

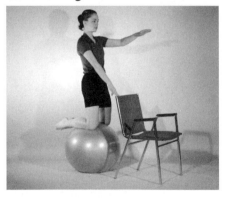

- one point of stable contact, eyes open
- contract and hold TrA

21   **Ball Kneeling**

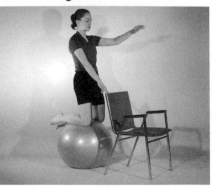

- one point of stable contact, eyes closed
- contract and hold TrA

Deep Layer / Position Sense Exercises

Progressing from easier to harder ... concentrate on maintaining a quality TrA contraction throughout and try to hold each posture a few seconds longer every day.

22   **Ball Kneeling**

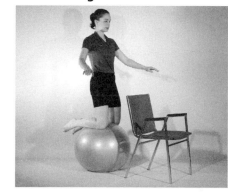

- no points of stable contact, eyes open
- contract and hold TrA

23   **Ball Kneeling**

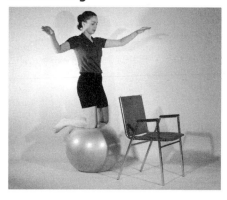

- no points of stable contact, eyes open, add arm movement
- contract and TrA

24   **Ball Kneeling**

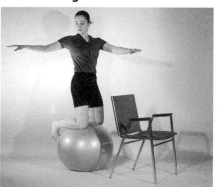

- no points of stable contact, eyes open, add trunk movement
- contract and hold TrA

Deep Layer / Position Sense Exercises

Progressing from easier to harder ... concentrate on maintaining a quality TrA contraction throughout and try to hold each posture a few seconds longer every day.

25   Ball Kneeling

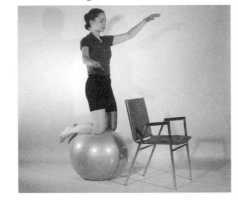

- no points of stable contact, eyes closed
- contract and hold TrA

26   Ball Kneeling

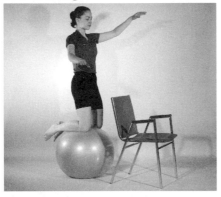

- no points of stable contact, eyes closed, with arm movements
- contract and hold TrA

27   Ball Standing

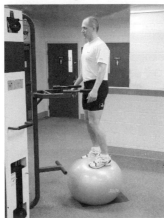

- from a safety perspective this is not an exercise for everyone

- **bones get broken, shoulders get dislocated and skulls get cracked open attempting this exercise**

- for a **very small percentage** of athletes, there is value in taking the deep layer exercises to this level

- the safest way to begin this exercise is to place the ball at the base of a tricep dip rack, as in the picture
- you may then lower yourself on to the ball, while keeping a handhold close by
- as you become more comfortable, take your hands off the bar for brief periods - a few seconds - until you develop a feel for the standing position

DO NOT ATTEMPT THIS WITHOUT A RELIABLE SPOTTER CLOSE BY AT ALL TIMES

Middle Layer Stabilization Exercises

The middle layer exercises are organized into three sections: transversus abdominis (TrA) exercises, static middle layer exercises and dynamic middle layer exercises. Within each section, all exercises progress from easier to harder. I would recommend developing good control of the TrA exercises before beginning the static exercises. Likewise, good command of the static exercises should precede beginning the dynamic exercises.

Transversus Abdominis

The beauty of these exercises is that they train the transversus abdominis in a very specific manner, essentially duplicating how the muscle functions in real life. TrA works to stabilize your trunk while your limbs are in motion (walking, throwing, paddling, running, reaching, lifting etc.)

1   Basic TrA activation

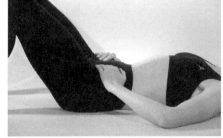

- contract pelvic floor (see instructions on pages 33 & 34) then ...
- draw in lower abdomen while breathing gently - think of:
    - ... creating a concave lower abdomen, or
    - ... pulling your belly button into your spine, or
    - ... pulling your lower abdomen away from the inside edge of your pants
- use your finger tips to monitor muscle contraction; fingers should be just inside the 'front corners' of your pelvis
- you should feel a small to moderate amount of tension develop under your finger tips as you contract your pelvic floor and transversus muscles
- *if you are doing this correctly, you should feel some amount of muscle soreness across your lower abdomen by the next day*

2   TrA with bent knee fall out

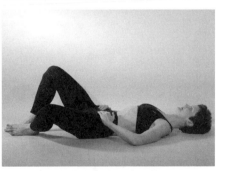

- maintain TrA contraction while letting knee move slowly outwards toward floor; alternate legs

* use your finger tips to monitor tension in the lower abdomen - if you feel this tension drop as you move your leg, do not move the leg further - only move your hip within a range of motion through which you can keep transversus contracted

3   TrA with heel slide

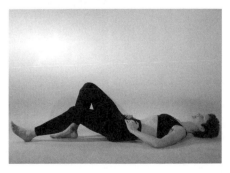

- maintain TrA contraction while sliding foot away slowly along floor; alternate legs

* same rules about hip movement and muscle tension in transversus - if you feel the tension drop, do not move the hip any further
- with practice you will be able to move the hip through full range while keeping transversus contracted

48

Middle Layer Stabilization Exercises
Transversus Abdominis

4   TrA with arms reaching over head

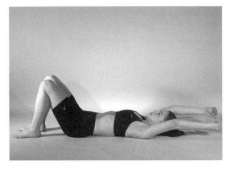

• maintain TrA contraction while letting arms move overhead toward floor

* if you feel the tension in your transversus drop as you move your arms, do not move further - only move your arms as far as you are able to keep your transversus contracted

5   TrA with single knee lift

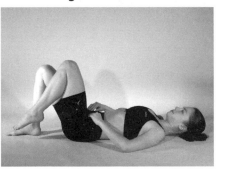

• maintain TrA contraction while lifting thigh toward your shoulder
• this is a difficult exercise ... it may take some practice to coordinate your pelvic floor and abdominal contractions with the thigh motion

* use your finger tips to monitor tension in the lower abdomen - if you feel this tension drop as you move your leg, do not move the leg further - move only so far as you can while maintaining a good contraction in transversus

6   TrA with single knee lift and opposite side bent knee fall out

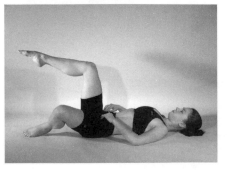

• maintain TrA contraction while lifting one thigh toward your shoulder while the other thigh moves outward toward the floor ... again, it may take some practice to coordinate your abdominal work with the thigh movements

* use your finger tips to monitor tension in the lower abdomen - if you feel this tension drop as you move your legs, do not move the legs further - move only so far as you can while maintaining a good contraction in transversus

Middle Layer Stabilization Exercises
Transversus Abdominis

7   **TrA with single knee lift and opposite arm overhead reach**

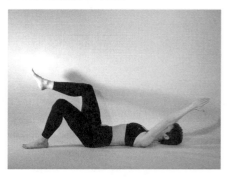

The 'dying bug' exercise ...

• maintain TrA contraction while letting arms move overhead toward floor
• not too difficult once you have mastered exercises 4 and 5

8   **TrA with double knee lift**

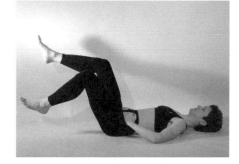

• maintain TrA contraction while lifting one leg up, then the other
• once both thighs are vertical, lower one leg then the other very slowly - concentrate on your transversus!

• for most people, the hard part with this exercise is maintaining a good TrA contraction as you are about to initiate movement in the *second* leg
• focus on your TrA contraction *not* the movement of the second leg

9   **TrA with single knee lift and opposite side leg extension**

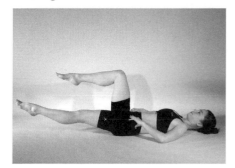

A very, very difficult exercise!

• most back pain patients find it very difficult to develop sufficient TrA strength and control to do this correctly and thus safely
• this exercise should therefore be done only on the advice of a physical therapist

Middle Layer Stabilization Exercises

Transversus Abdominis

10   **TrA with double leg lowering**

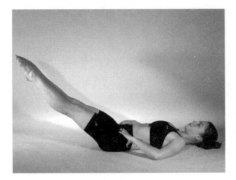

I hesitated about including this exercise because it is so incredibly demanding. Many, many people attempt this exercise but very few people - even elite athletes - can do this correctly and therefore safely.

Remember, if you are not maintaining a perfect TrA contraction this exercise has the potential to hurt your back more than help it.

• this exercise should therefore be done only on the advice of a physical therapist

Static Middle Layer Exercises

The following is a lengthy list of middle layer exercises, both static and dynamic. Your physiotherapist can help you make appropriate choices from this list based on your condition. Generally, most people will be working with two to six different middle layer exercises at any given time. As you develop greater core stability, you may try the more difficult exercises found toward the end of each section.

As with the deep layer exercises, maintain a consistent contraction in TrA while holding these postures. Initially try 5 - 10 repetitions, holding each for 5 - 10 seconds. As you get stronger, hold them longer (up to 30 or 45 seconds) but do fewer repetitions. Remember, correct technique is much more important than how long you can hold each posture and how many repetitions you can do. Never sacrifice quality for quantity.

1   Back Bridge - wide base of support, four points of stable contact

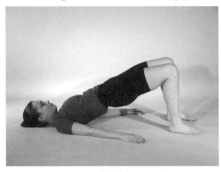

- establish a 'straight line' through your knee, hip and shoulder while contracting TrA

2   Back Bridge - wide base of support, two points of stable contact

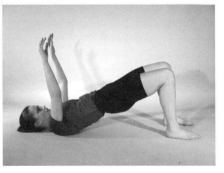

- establish a 'straight line' through your knee, hip and shoulder while contracting TrA

- in general, all the back-lying bridges place more emphasis on posterior muscles of the body such as our hamstrings, gluteals and latissimus

3   Back Bridge - narrow base of support, two points of stable contact

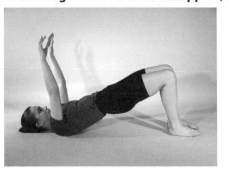

- establish a 'straight line' through your knee, hip and shoulder while contracting TrA
- your feet should be closer together than in the previous two exercises, but not touching
- allowing your inner thighs to touch leads to use of the inner thigh muscles to help stabilize the posture - occasionally a therapist may want you to do this, but usually it is a method of 'cheating'

Static Middle Layer Exercises

4   **Back Bridge - one point of stable contact**

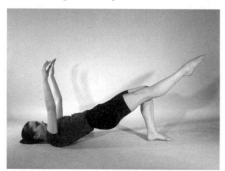

- maintain that 'straight line' through your knee, hip and shoulder while contracting TrA
- this is quite a lot more difficult than exercise 3 as it demands greater balance and strength

- initially, you may some develop some cramping in the back of your thigh since your buttocks and upper hamstrings must work in a shortened position to hold this posture ...
usually a simple hamstring stretch before and after is enough to solve this problem

5   **Back Bridge - two points of stable contact (feet on ball)**

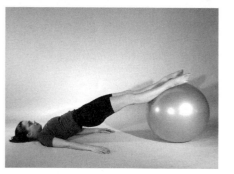

- maintain that 'straight line' through your knee, hip and shoulder while contracting TrA
- note that the hands are on the floor again to provide a stability assist now that you're using a ball

- less strength required to maintain the posture but obviously a greater stability and balance challenge

6   **Back Bridge - no points of stable contact (feet on ball)**

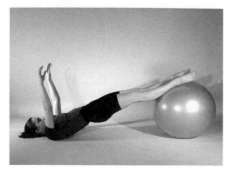

- maintain that 'straight line' through your knee, hip and shoulder while contracting TrA
- with the hands off the floor the trunk stability demand increases dramatically

- some people will move relatively quickly from exercise 5 to 6 while others will take longer to find their balance and trunk stability
- each time you add a level of stability challenge it becomes harder to maintain a good TrA contraction - work dilegently at this ... the TrA will give you the sense of stability you need to perform these more advanced exercises

Static Middle Layer Exercises

**7   Back Bridge - lying on ball, feet on floor;
two points of stable contact, wide base of support**

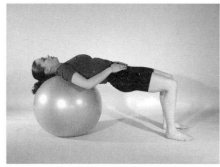

- maintain that 'straight line' through your knee, hip and shoulder while contracting TrA
- this is usually less challenging than exercise 6

- to get into this position, begin by sitting on the ball as in the exercises on page 31, then walk your feet away from the ball as you lie back
- note that your head and neck should rest comfortably on the ball - do not allow your head to remain unsupported

**8   Back Bridge - lying on ball, feet on floor;
two points of stable contact, narrow base of support**

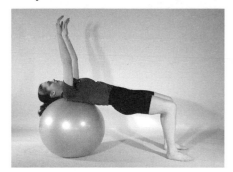

- maintain that 'straight line' through your knee, hip and shoulder while contracting TrA
- feet are closer together but not touching - keep the inner thighs apart too unless a therapist has instructed you to do so

- again, most people will find exercise 6 more challenging than this one

**9   Back Bridge - lying on ball, one foot on floor;
one point of stable contact**

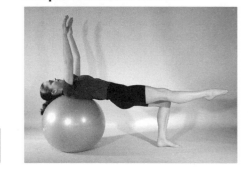

- maintain that 'straight line' through your knee, hip and shoulder while contracting TrA
- just as there was a big jump in difficulty from exercise 3 to 4, this exercise is much harder than exercise 8 ...add a hamstring stretch if neccessary

Static Middle Layer Exercises

Note: *Done under the supervision of a physical therapist, exercises 10 to 24 can also be very useful for people with shoulder instabilities.*

10   Front Bridge - from knees, four points of stable contact

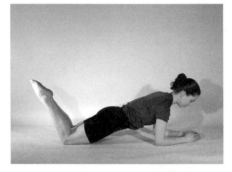

- maintain that 'straight line' through your knee, hip and shoulder *and neck* while contracting TrA
- in general, all the front-lying bridges place more emphasis or demand on the anterior muscles such as the abdominals, hip flexors and hip adductors (inner thigh)
- the front-lying exercises also place great demand on the shoulder girdle muscles - you must have sufficient shoulder strength to do many of the more advanced versions
- performing the exercises correctly will develop strength in your shoulder stabilizers as well as your trunk

11   Front Bridge - from toes, wide base of support, four points of stable contact

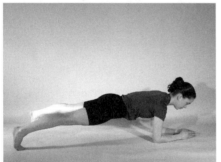

- maintain that 'straight line' through your knee, hip and shoulder and neck while contracting TrA

12   Front Bridge - from toes, narrow base of support, four points of stable contact

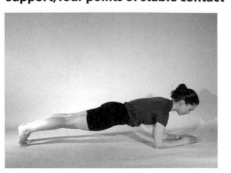

- maintain that 'straight line' through your knee, hip and shoulder and neck while contracting TrA
- recall that when beginning these 'static' or non-moving exercises, hold each for 5 to 10 seconds and work up to 10 repetitions
- when you can do 10, 10 second repetitions begin holding each repetition longer but do fewer of them
- eventually you will be holding each repetition for 20 to 45 seconds, but doing only 3 to 5 repetitions

Static Middle Layer Exercises

**13   Front Bridge - from toes,
three points of stable contact**

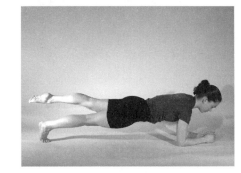

- maintain that 'straight line' through your knee, hip and shoulder and neck while contracting TrA

- usually much more demanding than exercises 11 or 12

**14   Front Bridge Walkout -
two points of stable contact, thighs on ball**

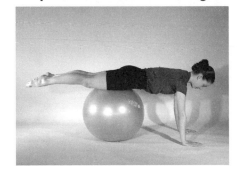

- begin by kneeling on the floor with the ball resting against your abdomen - then roll onto the ball and walk your hands forward
- maintain that 'straight line' through your knee, hip and shoulder and neck while contracting TrA

- the exercise is made more difficult by walking your hands further out and having the ball support you closer to your feet as in the next exercise

**15   Front Bridge Walkout -
two points of stable contact, feet on ball**

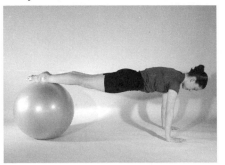

- maintain that 'straight line' through your ankle, knee, hip, shoulder and neck while contracting TrA

- as the unsupported length of your body increases, it becomes more difficult to keep TrA activated correctly - pay close attention to the contraction of TrA as you progress into these more difficult exercises

Static Middle Layer Exercises

16   **Front Bridge Walkout**
two points of stable contact, one foot on ball, lift other leg

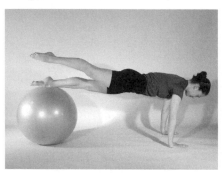

- maintain that 'straight line' through your ankle, knee, hip, shoulder and neck while contracting TrA

- quite difficult in terms of strength and balance
- these more advanced variations on the basic front bridge walkout can provide a great workout for the whole body but beware of the effect of muscle fatigue - stop when you feel your technique is suffering

17   **Front Bridge Arms on Ball 1 -**
two knees on floor, arms on ball

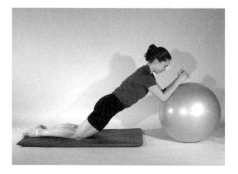

- maintain that 'straight line' through your knee, hip, shoulder and neck while contracting TrA

- exercises 17 - 18 are difficult primarily from a balance perspective and are thus effective deep and middle layer exercises

18   **Front Bridge Arms on Ball 2 -**
one knee on floor, arms on ball

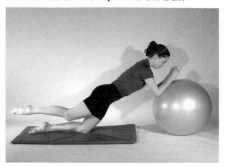

- very tricky to balance with this one!
- again, these are also excellent for people who require improved stabilization of their shoulder girdle

Static Middle Layer Exercises

19   **Front Bridge Arms on Ball 3**
two feet on floor, arms on ball

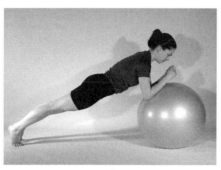

- maintain that 'straight line' through your ankle, knee, hip, shoulder and neck while contracting TrA

- difficult in terms of balance and strength - a lack of shoulder girdle and trunk strength often limit people's ability to do this exercise

20   **Front Bridge Arms on Ball 4**
one foot on floor, arms on ball

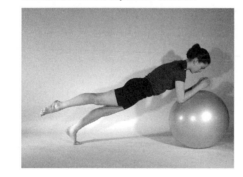

- maintain that 'straight line' through your ankle, knee, hip, shoulder and neck while contracting TrA

- our model has terrific shoulder girdle strength and a highly developed balance sense which she demonstrates here!

21   **Side Bridge - from knees**

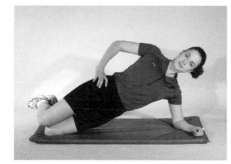

- even in the side position, maintain that 'straight line' through your knee, hip, shoulder and neck while contracting TrA

- these next exercises done in the side position target the lateral trunk muscles very effectively - expect some 'post-workout' muscle soreness the day after doing these for the first time

Static Middle Layer Exercises

22   **Side Bridge - from feet**

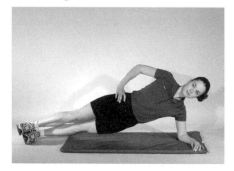

24   **Side Bridge - from feet, lift top leg**

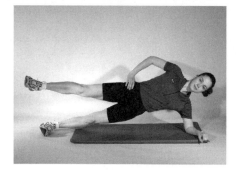

• a very difficult exercise!

Note to Therapists:
• correct performance of this requires excellent activation and strength in the weightbearing-side gluteus medius
• as the upper hip is abducted, a greater stabilization demand is placed on the weightbearing gluteus medius
• a good exercise to train the *transverse system* as per Diane Lee's /Andry Vleeming's 'Outer Unit'

Dynamic Middle Layer Exercises

Same instructions as per the static middle layer exercises - maintain TrA contraction and slowly increase the number of repetitions of each exercise. You must have excellent TrA control and the ability to hold most of the static middle layer exercises for 30 seconds before attempting these more difficult exercises.

NOTE: Start positions are on the left, finishing positions on the right.

1   **Back Bridge Hamstring Curl - feet on ball, curl knees toward chest; two points of stable contact**

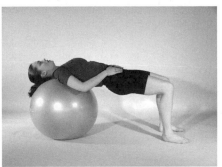 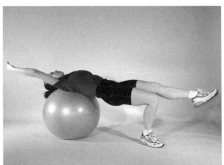

2   **Back Bridge Hamstring Curl - feet on ball, curl knees toward chest; no points of stable contact**

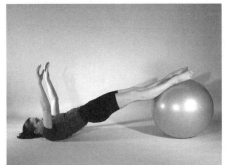 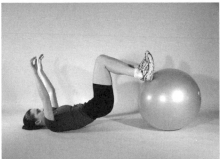

3   **Back Bridge 'Dying Bug' - feet on floor; slowly straighten one knee and opposite arm; one point of stable contact**

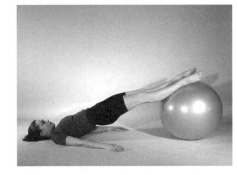 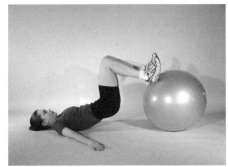

Dynamic Middle Layer Exercises

NOTE: Start positions are on the left, finishing positions on the right.

4   **Front Bridge Walkout & Leg Lift**
         • feet on ball, lift one leg off the ball then move it away from you and to the side (abduction)

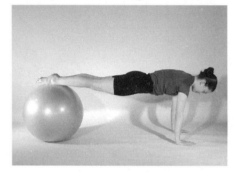 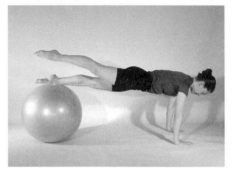

5   **Front Bridge Walkout, Knees to Chest**
         • feet on ball then slowly bring knees toward chest

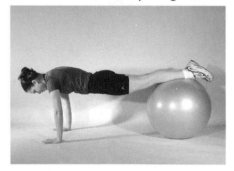 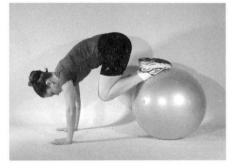

6   **Front Bridge Walkout, Pike**
         • feet on ball then slowly fold body at midsection (pike position)

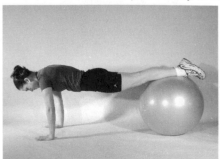 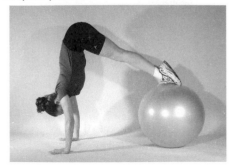

Dynamic Middle Layer Exercises

NOTE: Start positions are on the left, finishing positions on the right.

7   Front Bridge Walkout and Trunk Twist
· feet on ball; lift one leg, rotate body toward side of lifted leg - pelvis becomes vertical

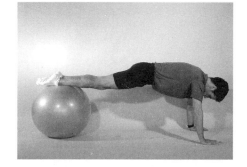
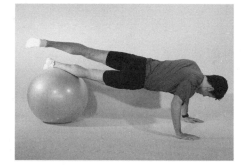

CAUTION!
Dynamic middle layer exercise number 8 is a very demanding trunk and shoulder girdle exercise.

However , it may cause severe shoulder damage if performed incorrectly. Do not over-extend your forward lean or reach - your shoulders must remain bent and must never be in a straight line with your body.

People who have dislocated their shoulder in the past or who have shoulder instability should not attempt this exercise.

---

8   Front Bridge Arms on Ball
· lean body forward and backward with arms supporting body weight on ball, both knees on floor

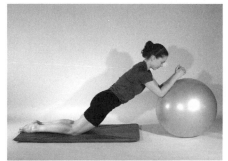
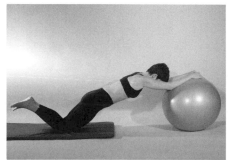

Outer Layer Exercises

Where indicated these exercises should be performed with a maintained TrA contraction. Remember that for most people the muscles associated with the deep and middle layer exercises are more important to train than these larger movement muscles. If you need extra strength in the large movement muscles of the trunk then include these in your program. You must have at least a moderate degree of trunk stabilization and good skill with various static and dynamic middle layer exercises before using these exercises in your program.

1   Abdominal Crunches

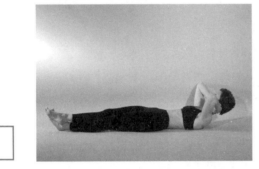

- potentially hard on the neck and will not directly stabilize the spine
- having strong outer layer abdominals may allow TrA to be more effective at stabilizing the spine

- *maintain a contraction in TrA and perform these with your legs straight*

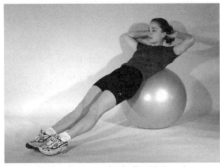

- may also be done on the ball with hands supporting your neck

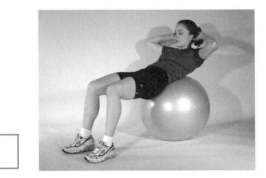

2   Opposite Arm & Leg Lift

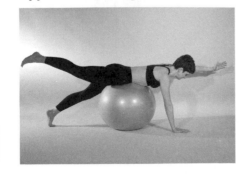

- works the large back extensor muscles
- *maintain contraction in TrA while extending opposite arm and leg; keep spine and pelvis level without twisting*

Outer Layer Exercises

3   Extensions

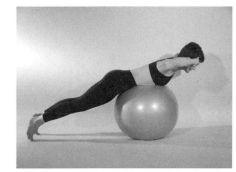

- requires a healthy back and good stabilization from the middle layers (TrA)
- maintain contraction in TrA
- lay face down on ball, with ball at or above waistline; raise trunk to the horizontal level and slowly lower

4   The Butt Buster

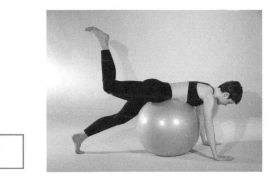

- maintain contraction in TrA
- focus on movement at the hip and stability or lack of movement at the lower back

Chapter 5
Sample Spinal Stabilization Programs

The following are samples only. They are provided only to illustrate a rational progression from beginner to advanced programs. Your program should reflect your injury, your stage of recovery and your stabilization ability. Always refer to the concepts discussed in chapter three when designing or progressing your program. If you have a back problem of any kind, a physical therapist should be consulted to help you select the most effective and safe options.

Please note that not all exercises are intended to be performed on a daily basis. You might use one or two exercises from each group (deep, middle and outer layers) on Monday and Thursday and a different exercise or two from the same groups on Tuesday and Friday. Mix up your program every few days to keep things interesting and keep your body challenged. Appreciate that you will have days where the exercises will seem easy and well controlled and others where you will struggle. This is normal. Over a period of a few weeks you will notice significant changes both in terms of your ability to perform the exercises but, more importantly, how well you feel.

Beginner Level

Maintain a correct TrA contraction with all exercises.

Deep Layer Exercises

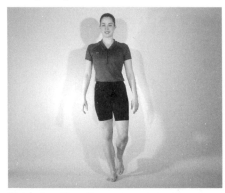

Single Leg Standing, eyes open

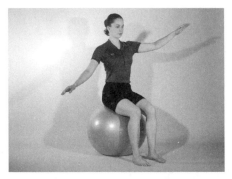

Ball Sitting, eyes open, with arm movement

Middle Layer Exercises

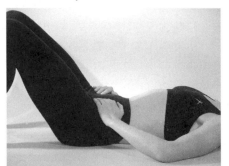

Basic TrA activation

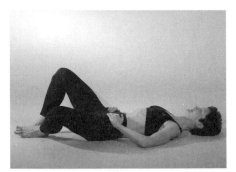

TrA with bent knee fall out

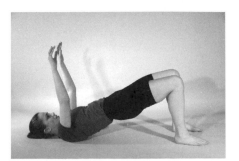

Back Bridge - wide base of support, two points of stable contact

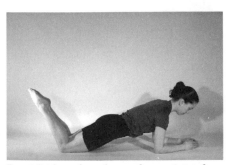

Front Bridge - from knees, four points of stable contact

Early Intermediate Level

Maintain a correct TrA contraction with all exercises.

Deep Layer Exercises

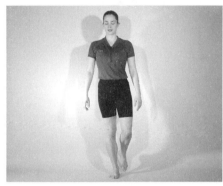

Single Leg Standing - eyes closed

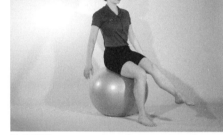

Ball Sitting - eyes closed, one point of stable contact

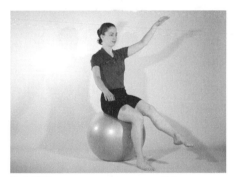

Ball Sitting - eyes open, one point of stable contact, with arm movements

Middle Layer Exercises

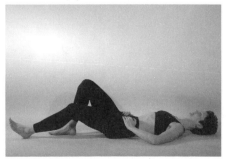

TrA with heel slide

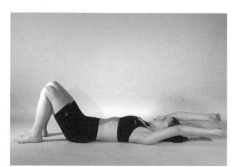

TrA with arms reaching overhead

Early Intermediate Level

Maintain correct TrA contraction with all exercises.

Middle Layer Exercises (continued)

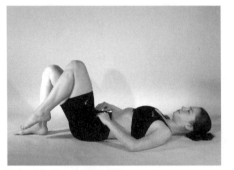

TrA with single knee lift

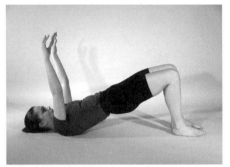

Back Bridge - narrow base of support, two points of contact

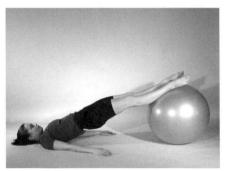

Back Bridge - two points of stable contact (feet on ball)

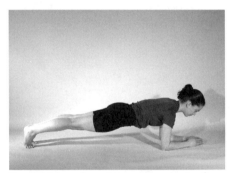

Front Bridge - from toes, narrow base of support, four points of stable contact

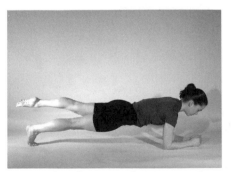

Front Bridge - from toes, three points of stable contact

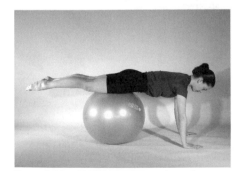

Front Bridge Walkout - two points of stable contact, thighs on ball

Late Intermediate Level

Maintain correct TrA contraction with all exercises.

Deep Layer Exercises

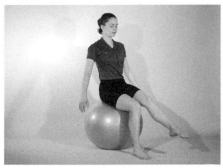

Ball Sitting - eyes closed, one point of stable contact

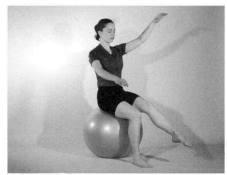

Ball Sitting - eyes closed, one point of stable contact, with arm movements

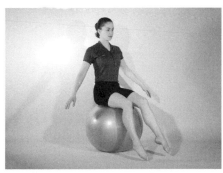

Ball Sitting - no points of stable contact

Middle Layer Exercises

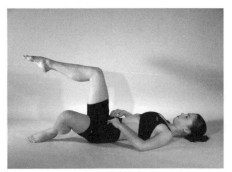

TrA with single knee lift and opposite side bent knee fall out

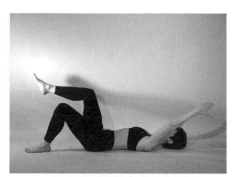

TrA with single knee lift and opposite arm overhead reach (the 'dying bug' exercise)

Late Intermediate Level

Maintain correct TrA contraction with all exercises.

Middle Layer Exercises (continued)

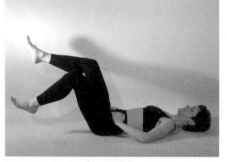

TrA with double knee lift

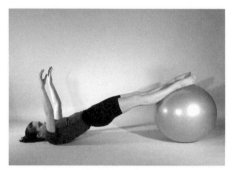

Back Bridge - no points of stable contact

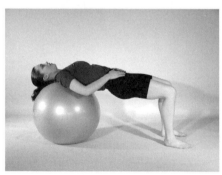

Back Bridge - lying on ball, feet on floor; two points of stable contact, wide base of support

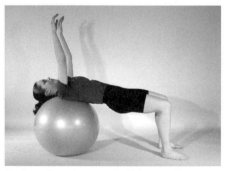

Back Bridge - lying on ball, feet on floor; two points of stable contact, narrow base of support

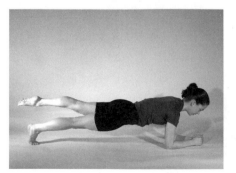

Front Bridge - from toes, three points of stable contact

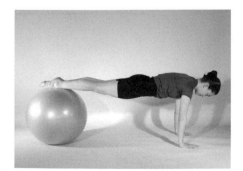

Front Bridge Walkout - two points of stable contact, feet on ball

Late Intermediate Level

Maintain correct TrA contraction with all exercises.

Middle Layer Exercises (continued)

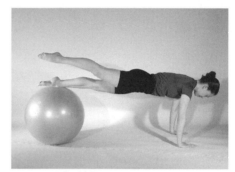

Back Bridge Hamstring Curl

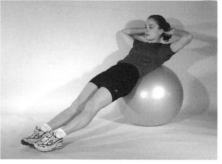

Front Bridge Walkout
- with leg lift

Outer Layer Exercises

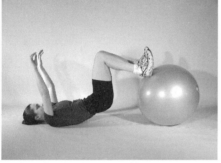

Side Bridge - from knees

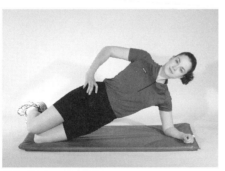

Abdominal Crunches

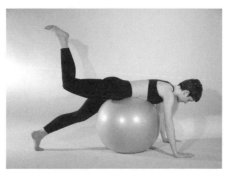

The Butt Buster
- front lying with knee bent

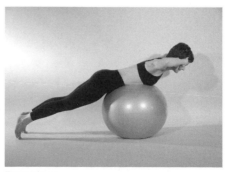

Extensions

Advanced Level

Maintain correct TrA contraction with all exercises.

Deep Layer Exercises

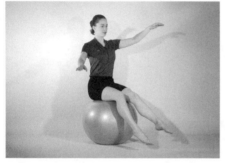

Ball Sitting - no point of stable contact, with arm movements

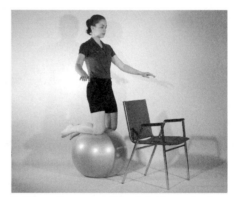

Ball Kneeling - no point of stable contact, eyes open

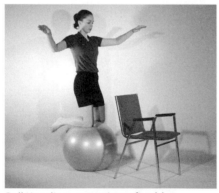

Ball Kneeling - no points of stable contact, eyes open, add arm movement

Middle Layer Exercises

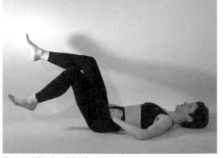

TrA with double knee lift

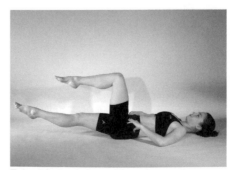

TrA with single knee lift and opposite side leg extension

Advanced Level

Maintain correct TrA contraction with all exercises.

Middle Layer Exercises (continued)

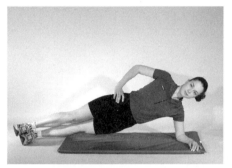

Side Bridge - from feet

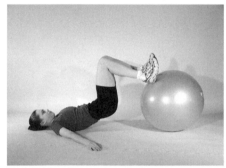

Back Bridge Hamstring Curl

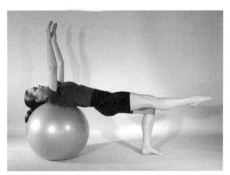

Back Bridge - single leg extension

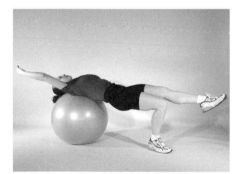

Back Bridge 'Dying Bug'

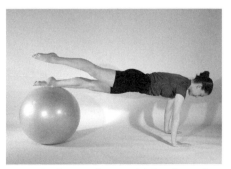

Front Bridge Walkout with backward
leg lift

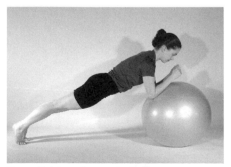

Front Bridge, Arms on Ball 3

Advanced Level

Maintain correct TrA contraction with all exercises.

Middle Layer Exercises (continued)

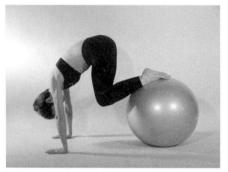

Front Walkout - Knee to Chest

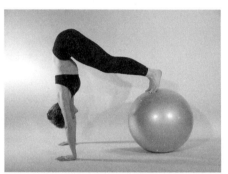

Front Walkout - Pike

Outer Layer Exercises

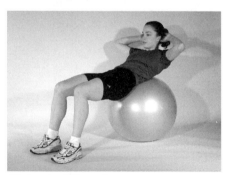

Abdominal Crunches

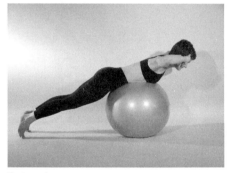

Extensions

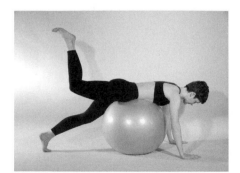

The Butt Buster

Olympic Level

Maintain correct TrA contraction with all exercises.

Deep Layer Exercises

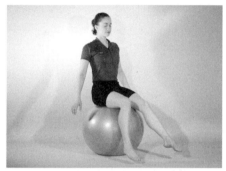

Ball Sitting - no point of stable contact

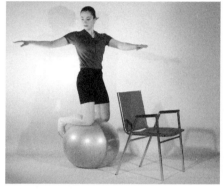

Ball Kneeling - no point of stable contact, add trunk movement

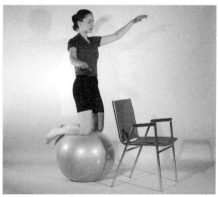

Ball Kneeling - no point of stable contact, eyes closed

Middle Layer Exercises

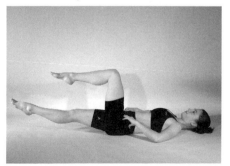

TrA with single knee lift and opposite side leg extension

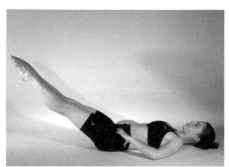

TrA with double leg lowering

Olympic Level

Maintain correct TrA contraction with all exercises.

Middle Layer Exercises (continued)

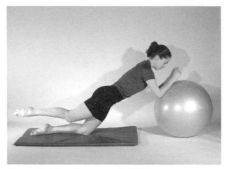

Front Bridge Arms on Ball 2 - one knee on floor, both arms on ball

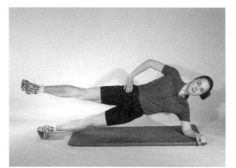

Side Bridge - from feet, lift top leg

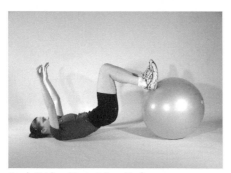

Back Bridge Hamstring Curl

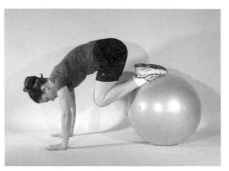

Front Bridge Walkout Knees to Chest

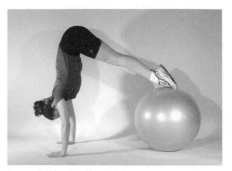

Front Bridge Walkout Pike

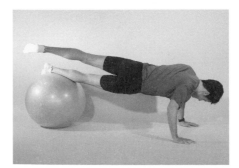

Front Bridge Walkout Trunk Twist

Olympic Level

Maintain correct TrA contraction with all exercises.

Outer Layer Exercises

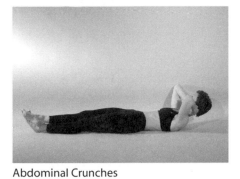

Abdominal Crunches

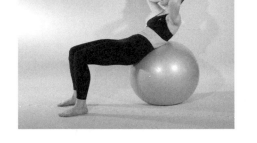

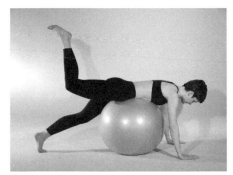

Extensions

The Butt Buster

Chapter 6
Stabilization Training and the Competitive Athlete

In the late 1950's and early 1960's, a Canadian physiologist, Hans Selye, developed what would become the single most important theory in sport conditioning science: The Specificity Principle of Training. This concept allowed sports conditioning specialists to design dramatically improved training programs for athletes of all kinds. Elegantly simple but truly fundamental to successful conditioning, the specificity principle states that *the human body will respond to any form of physical training in a highly predictable fashion.*

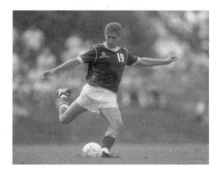

A person whose normal physical activity program includes four, 12 km runs per week will develop specific physiological adaptations over a relatively short period of time which will increase their aerobic capacity; however, they will not experience any significant increase in their muscle mass or strength as this involves the anaerobic side of their physiology. Likewise, the person who performs three strength training sessions per week will increase their anaerobic capacity (i.e., strength) but only in the specific muscles which have been trained. The person will not realize a similar scale increase in their aerobic fitness, and their strength gains will occur only in the muscles which have been targeted during their training sessions. In other words, whatever the human body does on a regular basis is exactly what the body will become *better* at doing on a regular basis.

This simple fact of human physiology has made it possible for strength and conditioning coaches to virtually guarantee sport performance improvements using appropriately designed exercise programs. The person who trains in a manner specific to their sport will experience physiologic adaptations which will lead to improved sport performance - guaranteed. It has to happen this way because that is how our body works.

This means, for example, that the person who runs 3 to 5 times each week at a moderate pace but for progressively longer periods of time will become better at long distance running; however, the flip side of the specificity principle reminds us that the person who runs long and slow will *not* become any better at sprinting. Training long and slow does not train the body for short and fast. Again, *the body responds to training in a very predictable fashion*. Our body's physical performance abilities (that is our aerobic, anaerobic, flexibility, agility and balance capabilities) will develop and improve, but only if we perform exercises which challenge each in a directed manner.

In the decades following the development of the specificity principle, sports conditioning has matured significantly. World records continue to be shattered in a variety of events and sports such as hockey are played by athletes who are remarkably faster and stronger than even 15 years ago. While the training of athletes has become more sophisticated over the past 40 years, one aspect of performance conditioning had remained overlooked until very recently.

If we consider the techniques used by most athletes to develop strength in their core and limbs, we will see that a majority of recreational and competitive athletes still perform exercises designed to isolate a muscle group and train it separately from the rest of the body. The athlete will lay or sit on a bench of some form (which supports and stabilizes their trunk) as they perform exercises which target their biceps, hamstrings, chest, etc.

This approach to strength training developed out of the body-building culture where the single objective of training is to build enormous amounts of muscle mass. A body-builder isn't especially concerned with applying that increased muscle mass to some functional activity; instead, their interest is limited to the aesthetics of large muscles. The problem with this approach to athletic conditioning, is that to some extent, it fails the training specificity test. There is no sport known to man where the athlete uses individual, isolated muscles in the performance of their sport. Tennis, golf, running, swimming, gymnastics, skiing, rowing, paddling, basketball, volleyball - all sports require the body to function as a *linked system* of muscles and joints.

This linked system of muscles and joints provides us with an important mechanical advantage; the transfer of energy from one part of the body to another. Virtually all sports movements depend on an efficient transfer of energy between the lower body and upper body. Sprinters generate some of their acceleration via their upper limbs while baseball pitchers develop higher throwing velocities through the kinetic energy developed in their legs. The trunk of course is the middle link in the chain, the segment through which this shared energy must pass. If the trunk is not stable, some of this energy is lost, requiring the limbs to work harder resulting in less efficient movement.

Some conditioning coaches, usually those of national team or professional athletes, recognized this deficit and have incorporated exercises such as squats and dead-lifts into their athlete's training programs. These require the body to function in a more realistic manner in that multiple muscles and joints are used in the execution of the exercise.

While these are an improvement over exercises which isolate a single muscle, they do not attend to the issues of core stability and position sense. The athlete is often expected to perform challenging and potentially dangerous exercises without first having developed an adequate degree of spinal stabilization.

In response to these concerns, some coaches will state that the traditional approach to training works just fine. They point to the increasingly faster times attained by world class athletes as proof that current approaches are sufficient. These coaches are, in part, correct. Current techniques are vastly superior to those used 30 or 40 years ago; however, current techniques are not as well refined as they could be. They are 'sufficient' only so long as the majority of athletes are using the same approach, creating something of a level, albeit handicapped, playing field. As long as all athletes train this way, they are all exposed to the same relative deficit in training and no single athlete will experience a significant disadvantage. The fact that stabilization training is a new concept should not prevent us from exploiting its benefits to further improve upon an already improved approach.

Training muscles in isolation (or, at best, in functional groups) and without regard for core stability and position sense, will result in muscles which function in isolation and in athletes who have the capacity to produce significant power in their limbs but who lack sufficient spinal stabilization to apply that power safely and effectively. Revisiting our analogy of driving blindfolded, the effect of this form of training is to place our blindfolded driver in a Formula One race car; the potential for damage is exponentially increased.

A bench should be something you rest on between shifts ...

All sports require the athlete's body to function in some form of *stability challenged* circumstance. Soccer, lacrosse, baseball, golf, running (distance or sprinting), all require the athlete to stabilize their body from within, that is, to use their body's stabilizing muscles to support their trunk, hips and shoulders during the activity. Sports such as hockey, rugby, dance, figure skating, soccer and gymnastics place enormous stabilization demands on the core due to the rapid changes of direction and the stopping and starting inherent in the sport.

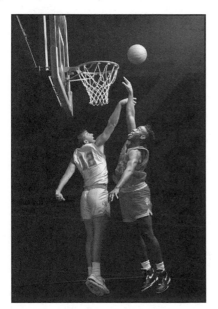

Skills such as swinging a baseball bat or a golf club, throwing a baseball or a football, performing a tumbling line in gymnastics, the accelerations involved in sprinting (either running, swimming or paddling) or the ability to absorb impact forces in hockey, rugby and basketball - all these create significant stabilization demands throughout the body. Even distance running requires the athlete's own muscles to support and stabilize their core over a single point of stable contact and a narrow base of support (their foot) approximately 180 times per minute.

Unfortunately, traditional strength training exercises are performed using a variety of artificial spinal stabilization aids - the benches and chairs which are designed to support or stabilize the athlete while they perform the exercise. These enable the athlete to isolate individual muscles as per the body-building approach to training. As discussed, there are drawbacks to this approach in that the athlete develops a somewhat unnatural form of strength, lacking coordination between core and limbs and lacking a well developed ability to stabilize the spine during activity.

The solution to this problem is quite simple: incorporate a degree of stability challenge into our traditional strength training exercises. By avoiding benches and chairs whenever possible the body is forced to create its own internal stabilization. Exercises that would normally have been done while standing with the feet shoulder width apart can be done standing on only one foot. Instead of using benches, use the large inflatable balls demonstrated in chapters four and five to sit, lie or lean on while doing any variety of 'traditional' strength exercises.

Making the transition from traditional to 'cutting edge' strength training ...

People who are just beginning a strength training program should begin training their core before training their arms and legs. In other words you should develop control in your deep and middle layers (as per chapters 3, 4 and 5) before moving to your outer layer. As your spinal stabilization skill develops then add any variety of outer layer exercises including traditional strength training exercises using machines such as Nautilus, Cybex, Keiser, or Atlantis.

Once you have developed good spinal stabilization skills and a moderate degree of outer layer strength via the machine-based exercises, it is time to begin learning how to use free weights. Having a qualified strength training specialist teach you correct and safe techniques when moving to free weights is a sound idea.

The final step is to combine your free weight and spinal stabilization training. This is accomplished by replacing benches and chairs with SwissBalls whenever possible. Initially, you may need to reduce the amount of weight used during the exercises as you incorporate the additional stabilization challenge into your exercise routine. This shouldn't be a concern in that, even though the amount of weight you're lifting may decrease somewhat, you are actually developing a greater degree of *functional* strength.

For those of you experienced with free weight training, continue as you have but begin working through the deep and middle layer exercises as presented in chapters 3, 4 and 5. Once you have developed good spinal stabilization skills and are comfortable doing at least the moderately challenging dynamic middle layer exercises, combine the two and replace your benches with SwissBalls. If you are a competitive athlete (and remember that even recreational athletes are often quite competitive) discuss the design of your program with a qualified strength training specialist. Remember that runners will need different strength programs than rowers, and gymnasts will need different programs than hockey players. The concept of stabilization-based strength training applies to all athletes but the actual program specifics will vary between different sports and between athletes.

Practical Tips:

Use a burst resistant ball for all your training.

All SwissBalls are not created equal. All have the potential to be punctured, some more easily than others. The key is to purchase a ball which will deflate slowly if it does develop a hole. Non burst-resistant balls can deflate in a split second, sending you crashing to the ground. If you happened to be doing an exercise involving free-weights you might be severely injured as the ball collapses. Expect to pay between $40.00 and $70.00 for a good quality, burst-resistant ball.

How big should the ball be?

This is not as cut and dry as some people would have you believe. The common answer to this question is that the ball should be of the correct size to allow your hips and knees to be at 90 degree angles when you sit on the ball. This is important if you are going to use the ball primarily for sitting. If you are going to use it for a variety of exercises, the size issue becomes a little more cloudy.

For example, when laying on the ball to perform a bench press, your arms should remain unsupported at the bottom of the movement. Larger balls will be wide enough to support your arms at the bottom, making the exercise somewhat easier. On the other hand, larger balls will be best for exercises involving kneeling or even (yikes!) standing on the ball. The best answer to the size question probably involves trying different size balls for a variety of exercises and determining which size will best meet your needs. A further complicating factor is that for some reason, sizing can be variable from one manufacturer to the next (that is, a 55 cm ball made by company A might be the same size as a 65 cm ball made by company B). In fact, size can vary between models made by the same company. Be prepared to experiment and perhaps return a ball that doesn't suit your size needs.

How much should the ball be inflated?

Again this is not easily defined. Softer, less inflated balls will have a larger surface or contact area with the floor and thus will be less 'tippy'. This might be a good thing for novices or people with especially poor balance reactions. More experienced users often want the added instability that comes with a maximally inflated ball. You can also think about varying the inflation of your ball depending on your skill level with certain exercises. For example if you have just begun the dynamic middle layer exercises and are having difficulty maintaining your balance, you might want to deflate your ball a little, making it more stable. As you get more comfortable with the exercises, inflate the ball further which will make the exercises more challenging. Experienced users tend to prefer a very firm ball as it is more responsive and demanding from a control perspective.

How many repetitions should I do?

If you are doing the spinal stabilization exercises as in chapters 3, 4 and 5 then you should perform each exercise to the point of fatigue. By fatigue I mean *the point at which you can no longer perform the exercise with excellent technique.* If you are doing stabilization-based strength training exercises such as chest presses or single arm rowing using the ball as a bench, select the number of repetitions as you would with traditional strength training exercises (lower weights and higher repetitions for muscular endurance, heavier weights and lower repetitions for strength and power development). You must be able to complete the set using good technique and while maintaining excellent spinal stabilization.

The following is a selection of stabilization-based strength exercises to demonstrate the potential application of these ideas. Have fun and at all times, be safe!

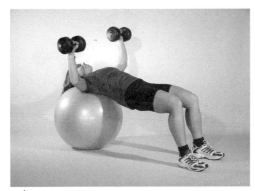
• chest press

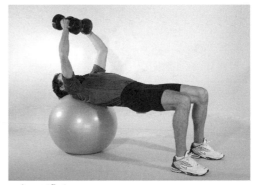
• chest 'fly'

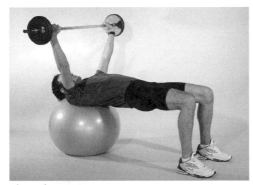
• bench press

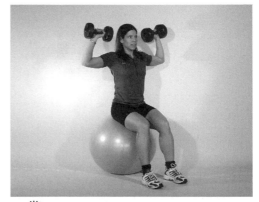
• military press

Strength Training Exercises Modified for Maximal Stabilization Challenge

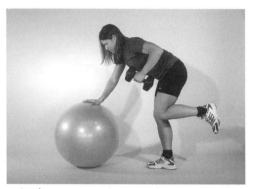

• single arm row

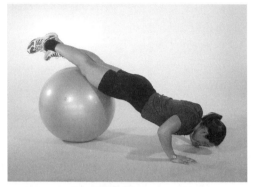

• push ups, from thighs

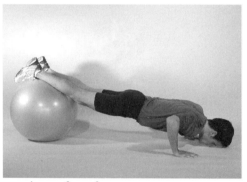

• push ups, from feet

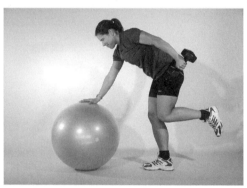

• single arm triceps press

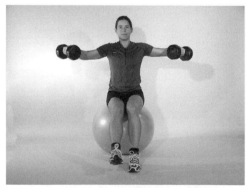

• shoulder abduction - sitting on ball, 1 point of stable contact

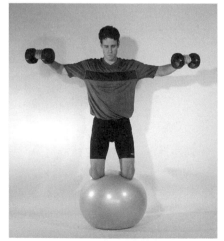

• shoulder abduction - kneeling on ball

Strength Training Exercises Modified for Maximal Stabilization Challenge

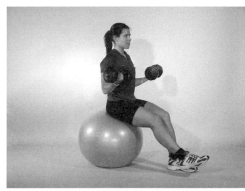

• seated bicep curl, 1 point of stable contact

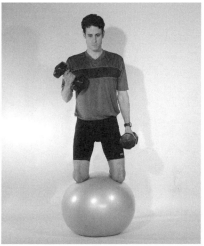

• kneeling bicep curl

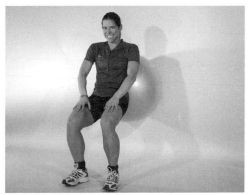

• ball on the wall squats

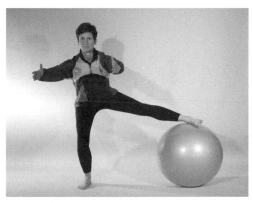

• single leg ball squats

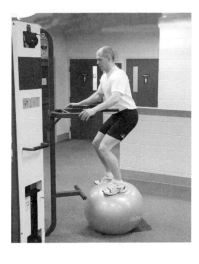

• ball squats - use tricep dip rack for safety!

Chapter 7
Spinal Stabilization in Back Injury Prevention Programs

In 1997 our facility was approached by a local health care complex to develop a back injury prevention program for its staff. We looked at the available research into existing back injury prevention programs and found a substantial number of studies. The majority of the studies which evaluated the effectiveness of these programs came to the same conclusion: back injury prevention programs hadn't worked. It appeared that programs which taught basic back strengthening exercises and lifting techniques failed to reduce the number of injuries, the severity of injuries or the number of days people lost at work due to back injury.

With our current understanding of spinal function we can identify two primary problems which existed with these programs. The strengthening exercises did not train the correct muscles (especially the deep and middle layers) and the lifting styles which were taught were not techniques the workers could actually use in their real-life jobs.

The exercise approach used in these programs was not based on the research described in this book; therefore, like all exercise-based programs of that era, success was limited by a relatively poor understanding of spinal function. The muscles targeted were typically from the outer layer and, as we have outlined previously, these muscles are not designed to protect and support our spine.

A related issue involved the use of the 'pelvic tilt' in old-style back education programs. The pelvic tilt was often described as a good posture to work from; indeed, many abdominal and other exercises emphasized this flexed position of the lower back. Further, many people were taught to lift while maintaining a pelvic tilt. Research in the mid-1990's demonstrated that the posture of the typical pelvic tilt actually leads to a loss of stability in the lower spine, as opposed to an increase in strength.

For this reason, the pelvic tilt is no longer used by most physiotherapists, except with people who have very specific types of back problems which still benefit from this posture. In general, the pelvic tilt should be avoided. It is now understood that maintaining a neutral low back posture, i.e., maintaining the natural curve of your lower back, is a much better posture to work from. This is true both for lifting and performing your core stabilization exercises.

A second problem with traditional back education/injury prevention programs centered on the ability for workers to actually use the lifting techniques taught to them. The lifting techniques taught on these courses were often not valid in the person's actual work environment. Clients have mentioned repeatedly that while they could easily perform a 'proper' lift in a practice situation, their ability to use these lifting styles on the job was minimal. Too often something about their work environment prevented them from using the 'ideal' style of lifting.

Examples of this are the night shift nurse who finds herself working alone instead of with a partner and putting 25 nursing home residents to bed without help; the long haul trucker who sits for ten hours behind the wheel, then has to unload a tightly packed truck without sufficient room to move about or lift correctly; the factory worker on an assembly line who performs the same repetitive body motion for two hours then needs to lift a single heavy item while rotating and bending forward.

In these circumstances, if the nurse, trucker or factory worker lacked the ability to stabilize their spine via their middle layer muscles, they would be exposed to an increased risk of spinal injury. Since these problems occur with regularity, and since our work environments can change suddenly and unpredictably, the only sensible solution is to recognize the need for people to have stronger stabilization muscles. If injury prevention programs continue to rely on the use of 'correct' lifting technique, people will continue to sustain back injuries. People must develop stronger, better stabilized spines if we are to truly decrease injury rates.

Another problem which may have affected the success of these and other programs was the extent to which the person performed their exercises. The best injury prevention program in the world will obviously fail if the person does not do the exercises. In the case of the older-style exercise programs, it is possible that people sensed the lack of true benefit of the exercises and were therefore not especially motivated to continue. Similarly, people may have been 'put off' the overall program, including their exercises, due to an awareness that they would never be able to lift at work in the style they were being taught on the back education course.

The bottom line with work-related back injury is that most people with physically demanding jobs lack the necessary core strength to do their job safely. The physical demands of working and lifting all day overwhelm their back's ability to correctly stabilize itself, leaving them vulnerable to injury. While correct lifting technique is certainly important and should be used whenever possible, the reality is that a person will occasionally be unable to lift properly. It is at these times that they must have adequate stabilization to lessen their risk of injury.

For these reasons, successful back injury prevention programs will no doubt begin to borrow from the spinal stabilization exercise catalogue. Given that spinal stabilization is based upon a more sophisticated appreciation of spinal function than were the older programs, this approach will be of benefit to virtually anyone who has a spine. The progression of exercises developed in chapters 3, 4 and 5 may be used for back injury prevention programs, just as it can be used for people recovering from back injury.

Chapter 8
Spinal Stabilization Success Stories

Many back exercise programs have been promoted in the past and this is obviously not the first time a health care professional has suggested that a certain exercise program would be of significant benefit to people with low back pain. While I hope that the explanations and arguments I have presented in favour of a trunk stabilization approach have been convincing, it is certainly reassuring to learn about others with similar problems who have benefited from this approach.

This section will introduce six people who, like you, have been through some kind of back pain problem. I have selected their stories because they represent a range of ages and fitness levels as well as different types of back pain; some of them sustained an injury to their spine while some simply developed a painful back for no apparent reason. Some of these people are competitive athletes, most are not.

The common denominator tying these people together however was their motivation to get well. They worked diligently and carefully at their exercises. Despite busy lives and hectic schedules they set aside time each week and did their exercises regularly. They made an effort to do the exercises with excellent technique. Each one of them will tell you that learning the transversus abdominis activation was difficult. Some people 'got it' in a few days, some took up to two weeks.

Despite the scheduling difficulties and the initial challenge of learning the transversus abdominis activation, they worked at their program. They no longer wanted to be limited by pain and they sensed the inherent logic in the design of the exercises. They recognized that this program was different; that *it made sense*.

Success Story 1

Bep Hardy-Mattern
- 40 years old; married with teenage children; teaches school
- enjoys walking for fitness
- many years of chronic low back pain with several unsuccessful attempts at rehabilitation

We were able to determine that Bep had an unstable sacroiliac joint. After years of joint instability and pain, her trunk muscles had virtually no idea of how to stabilize her low back and pelvis and she was in constant and severe pain. It was decided we would combine the use of a stabilizing belt designed for this injury as well as begin a trunk muscle stabilization program.

Bep's story ...

"It is very difficult to accept that your body is longer doing what it is supposed to. After close to thirty years of competitive field hockey, three children and a very active lifestyle, I was dealing with chronic problems with my back. The process started while I was pregnant with my first baby fifteen years ago and tried to lift a box full of books. From then on, my back would 'go out' at the slightest wrong move, rendering me helpless for a few weeks.

"Physiotherapy was helpful in getting me back on my feet, but I was starting to develop a weakness in my pelvic area and pain in my hips while going for short walks. It was clear that more was going on, but it took four different physiotherapists, two doctors and a lot of frustration on my part, before it became clear that 'loose' sacroiliac joints, caused by a combination of heredity, competitive sports, three babies in five years and a very active lifestyle, were the cause of my pain.

"Since being diagnosed with hypermobile sacroiliac joints I have faithfully done my strengthening exercises. I have to wear a support belt (try to explain this to Canada Customs when you travel!) but I am able to walk without pain, ski and be involved in any low impact activity I choose. I have to be careful to pay attention to my body and not overdo it, but the targeted strengthening exercises have allowed me to live an active, pain-free life again.

"While there are days when it is difficult to make time for the strengthening program, pain is a great motivator, and after having dealt with all the problems, the commitment is only a minor inconvenience and it comes with a great pay-off. In the future I would like to be strong enough to live without the belt. In the meantime I will continue with my training program and will return to my physiotherapist every few months to update and progress my training program."

Bep Hardy-Mattern

Success Story 2

Bruce Miller
- 42 years old; married; works as an occupational therapy assistant
- enjoys fitness walks and bike riding to and from work each day
- several years chronic low back pain due to a spondylolithesis (see chapter 2)

Bruce's condition is a classic form of joint instability - his joint injury leads to a progressive weakening of the trunk stabilization muscles. As these muscles get weaker, his back pain worsens. Since pain can also weaken or *inhibit* stabilization muscles, as his pain got worse his stabilization muscles became weaker yet.

Bruces's story ...

"My name is Bruce Miller and I had lower back pain along with pain and numbness that radiated down my right hip and leg. I had gained some weight and was frustrated with my physical condition. I was not able to walk around the block without having pain. I wanted to get back into shape so the first step that I took was to go see my doctor. He sent me for x-rays which showed that I had what is called a *spondylolithesis*, a big word for the lower back pain I was having. My doctor suggested that I see a physiotherapist.

"After an initial assessment by the physiotherapist a treatment program was set up. This consisted of exercises to strengthen the muscles in my abdomen which connect around to my lower back and help to stabilize my lower back. When I was first given the exercises I did them for a while but did not do them on a regular basis. My back felt better but I stopped. After a couple of months I returned to the physiotherapist who assessed my back and again made the recommendation to do the stabilization exercises.

"This time, I was more committed to doing the exercises as recommended by the physiotherapist. I worked hard at the exercises and kept regular appointments with the physiotherapist to monitor my progress. After a couple of months of regular stabilization exercises I was becoming pain free. I had very little back discomfort and the hip and leg problems were almost gone.

" I am able to do regular activity, ride my bike to work and have even participated in a 'mini triathalon'. I believe that it was the performance of the specific exercises that helped me to be pain free. I continue to do the exercises and would encourage you to follow the recommended program - it really does work!"

Bruce Miller

Success Story 3

Debbie Ling   • 23 years old, recently married; works as an occupational therapist
            • runs for fitness
            • chronic non-specific low back pain

Debbie had a localized increase in spinal joint motion at a single level of her lower back, a hypermobility. Specifically, her 4th and 5th lumbar vertebrae were 'loose' into forward bending. There had been no history of injury or trauma; however, for reasons unknown, her lumbar spine was not doing a good job of stabilizing itself. When she came to see me initially she had been unable to run for several weeks due to low back pain and her back was beginning to bother her with other activities as well, including her work.

Debbie's story ...

"Due to the hypermobility of my L4 and L5 vertebrae, I was experiencing back pain, most significantly after running several days in a row. When I went to see Mr. Jemmett at Maritime Physiotherapy, I was introduced to the trunk stabilization program as a way to strengthen the muscles around my 'loose' vertebrae. It was a concept that was very easy to understand, thus making it easy to incorporate the exercise program into my daily activities.

"Foremost, I could feel changes in how my back and overall trunk felt within a few weeks of doing the transversus abdominis exercises and progressing to the dynamic middle layer exercises. When I began to run again, I noticed an increase in the amount of strength in my abdominal, oblique and lower back muscles. Since then, my back continues to feel stronger and I don't experience back pain after running, as long as I maintain my exercise routine. Presently, I do my trunk stabilization exercises once per day, five to seven days per week.

"In addition to the benefits I've noticed with my running, other activities such as my work, as well as other sports such as swimming have been more comfortable too."

Debbie Ling

Success Story 4

Anne-Marie Wong

- 35 years old, married with young children; homemaker
- former gymnast, but hadn't exercised regularly for several years
- chronic non-specific low back pain

Anne Marie's problem was a generalized increase in spinal motion, most likely due to her years of training as a gymnast. As a teenager training for her sport, her young spine became more and more mobile. This would have occurred as the spinal ligaments became progressively longer and longer, allowing more and more joint motion to occur. This excess joint motion allowed her to move into positions most of us would never even think of attempting. Once the ligaments of a joint become loose, either by injury or activities such as gymnastics, they tend to stay loose. Therefore by the age of 35 she had excess spinal joint motion, but poor trunk muscle strength.

Anne Marie's story ...

"I had been suffering from increasingly chronic, non-specific back pain for approximately three years before I sought physiotherapy treatment. I had attributed my back pain to "getting old" but knew I should be exercising more. With my competitive rhythmic gymnastics background and its emphasis on range of motion far beyond the norm, I had assumed my problems were due to loss of flexibility. Thus I undertook a stretching program on my own. Needless to say, this did not alleviate my pain! I tried unsuccessfully to strengthen my abdominal muscles by performing 'crunch-type' exercises but would experience rather intense back pain. I knew I had to find help when even simple physical activities were causing me a great deal of discomfort.

"I experienced positive results with the trunk stabilization program almost immediately. I realized only after I began the program that my chronic pain had progressively been impacting on my life, both physically and emotionally. My back pain had been interfering with my sleep, which affected my mood and energy levels during the day. As my trunk strength improved it was as if a veil had been lifted. My pain level decreased dramatically as I progressed through the program. I began sleeping better, which in turn meant I had more energy during the day. I soon had the desire to begin an overall exercise program. I am now exercising regularly and feel better than I have in years. I have found the trunk stabilization exercise program to be extremely effective and the key component in resolving my back pain. The exercises are challenging as well as fun – not many exercise programs can make that claim! This program literally changed my life!"

Ann Marie Wong

Success Story 5

Chris Myers
• 33 years old, married with young children
• owns his own business and plays provincial level rugby
• came to see me several months following lumbar disc injury

Chris became my patient several months following his injury. While his pain had improved, he didn't feel strong enough to resume competitive rugby and was considering retiring from the sport.

Chris' Story ...

"I had a general lack of confidence that the disc was healed which resulted in two main problems: poor flexibilty due to the fear of injury from pushing my range of motion and a lack of core power due to no core specific activity or training.

"I had wanted to play rugby but was determined not to go through such an acute injury again. In fact I was discouraged by the othopaedic surgeon who had diagnosed my injury from ever playing contact sports again.

"I first went to see Rick prior to being asked to play in local play-offs and he thought I would be OK to play in a few weeks with the right training. This precluded me from the play-offs that season but I took his recommendations and started a core-specific exercise program. Within a month I did feel significantly better. I started out with very basic abdominal and lowerback exersises focusing on deep muscle control. As I got stronger I started to increase frequencies and levels of difficulty. Within 6 weeks I did feel like I was ready to play. Not leaving anything to chance, prior to playing I was examined by an orthopaedic surgeon and was given the OK to go ahead.

"Since then I have had two very successful rugby seasons at both the provincial and international levels. I am now a firm believer in core stabilty and incorporate elements of its principals in all of my training mainly through the the use of Swiss Balls and wobble boards."

Chris Myers

Success Story 6

Maggie Rossiter
- 47 years old, married with four children, aged 12 to 22
- works as a nurse
- began training for competitive sprint kayak paddling in the fall of 1999

Maggie had come to me for treatment of some shoulder and elbow problems that she felt were related to her new sport of sprint kayaking. She had begun her on-water training and shortly thereafter developed shoulder and elbow pain which always seemed worse after paddling. In the course of treating her arm problems, we began talking about her conditioning program. I suggested to her that there were a few things she might want to do differently, and she decided to have me develop her 'dry-land' training program for the ten months leading up to the Canadian National Paddling Championships in 2000.

Maggie's Story ...

"When Rick first discussed the concept of trunk stabilization training with me, it sounded as though this approach to conditioning had been tailor made for kayak racing. He described a conditioning program which would duplicate the lack of stability I experienced when paddling a racing kayak. By doing my dry-land training in this unstable manner, he felt that my body would learn to deal more effectively with the instability of my boat.

"The instability or 'tippy-ness' one experiences in a racing kayak is much like you would expect if you were asked to sit on a long pencil with your feet perched toward the tip and your behind toward the eraser. From this precarious position, you must develop huge amounts of power while at the same time maintaining your balance.

"Although many people see sprint kayaking as an upper body sport, the truth is that our power originates in the legs. This requires the trunk to transmit the power developed in the legs to the shoulders and arms and finally to the paddle. This 'unbroken transmission' of strength from the legs, through the trunk and finally to the upper body improved tremendously in my case after several weeks of stability training.

"The incorporation of the transversus abdominus activation was definitely an assest to me in my training program. The swissball and wobble board exercises were a welcome break from conventional training since an element of fun always existed. The strength training and core work that I did on the SwissBall were completely analogous to the stability challenges of paddling."

Maggie Rossiter

Success Stories Summary

Ultimately, the success of any one person's rehabilitation program is dependent on three factors; the degree of injury to the spine; the correctness of their exercise plan and the extent to which the person is motivated to get better. The science of spinal function is now mature enough for us to state that programs based on stabilization concepts offer the best non-surgical, non-pharmacologic solution to low back pain. From there, it is up to each of us to find ways to fit the exercises into our already busy lives and perform them as well as we can.

The stories these people have told certainly do not represent any form of valid scientific study. We cannot state categorically at this time that all people with spinal problems will realize the kind of significant improvements these people have. The intent of this section is to illustrate the fact that stabilization training has the potential to make significant changes in the way the spine functions and, in so doing, decrease a person's low back pain and/or improve their athletic performance.

Further we must recognize that stabilization training will not be the primary solution for all spinal problems. Some patients will need an operation to relieve the pressure placed on the nerves in their lower spine by a herniated disc. People with spinal stenosis will not likely see dramatic changes in their symptoms with stabilization training due to the nature of their spinal problem. Further, the extent to which people will fully recover is dependent on the degree of injury or damage to their spine. Bep Hardy continues to have some pain and finds there are still days where she needs to use her external stabilization belt.

Like all forms of medical treatment, spinal stabilization training will work best with certain forms of spinal problems. Fortunately the range of spinal problems which we can realistically expect to benefit from this approach is quite large. At some *appropriate* point in the recovery process, trunk stabilization exercises will be of benefit to the majority of people with back pain.

Appendix
References & Source Material

The following research articles and texts were used in the development of this text. Most of the articles pertain directly to spinal anatomy, biomechanics, motor control or spinal pathology. Others relate to stabilization or motor control issues in general or with regard to peripheral joints such as the shoulder or the knee.

Research Articles

Akiyama K, Takakura Y, Tomita Y, Sugimoto K, Tanaka Y, Tamai S; Neurohistology of the Sinus Tarsi and Sinus Tarsi Syndrome. J Orthop Science 1999 (4) 4: 299 - 303

deAndrade JR, Grant C, Dixon AJ; Joint Distension and Reflex Muscle Inhibition in the Knee. J Bone Joint Surg 1965 (47A) 2: 313 - 322

Beynnon BD, Johnson RJ, Fleming BC, Stankewich CJ, Renstrom PA; The strain behaviour of the anterior cruciate ligament during squatting and active flexion-extension. A comparison of an open and a closed kinetic chain exercise. Am J Sports Med 1997 (25) 6: 823 - 829

Blasier RB, Carpenter JE, Huston LJ; Shoulder proprioception. Effect of joint laxity, joint position and direction of motion. Orthop Rev 1994 (23) 1: 45 - 50

Brumagne S, Cordo P, Lysens R, Verschueren S, Swinnen S; The Role of Paraspinal Muscle Spindles in Lumbosacral Position Sense in Individuals with and without Low Back Pain. Spine 2000 (25) 8: 989-994

Carpenter JE, Blasier RB, Pellizzon GG; The effects of muscle fatigue on shoulder joint position sense. Am J Sports Med 1998 (26) 2: 262 - 265

Cresswell AG, Grundstrom H, Thorstensson A; Observations on intra-abdominal pressure and patterns of abdominal intra-muscular activity in man. Acta Physiol Scand 1992 (144): 409 - 418

Cresswell AG, Oddsson L, Thorstensson H; The influence of sudden perturbations on trunk muscle activity and intra-abdominal pressure while standing. Exp Brain Res 1994 (98): 336 - 341

Cholewicki J, Panjabi M, Khachatryan A; Stabilizing Function of Trunk Flexor-Extensor Muscles Around a Neutral Spine Posture. Spine 1997 (22) 19: 2207 - 2212

Crisco JJ, Panjabi MM; The Intersegmental and Multisegmental Muscles of the Lumbar Spine. Spine 1991 (16) 16: 793 - 799

Cuddeford T, Williams AK, Medeiros JM; Electromyographic Activity of the Vastus Medialis Oblique and Vastus Lateralis Muscles During Selected Exercises. J Manual Manip Ther 1996 (4) 1: 10 - 15

Danielsen JM, Johnsen R, Kibsgaard SK, Hellevik E; Early Aggressive Exercise for Postoperative Rehabilitation After Discectomy. Spine 2000 (25) 8: 1015 - 1020

Del Valle ME, Harwin SF, Maestro A, Murcia A, Vega JA; Immunohistochemical Analysis of Mechanoreceptors in the Human Posterior Cruciate Ligament: A Demonstration of its Proprioceptive Role and Clinical Relevance. J Arthroplasty 1998 (13) 8: 916 - 922

Escamilla RF, Fleisig GS, Zheng N, Barrentine SW, Wilk KE, Andrews JR; Biomechanics of the knee during closed and open kinetic chain exercises. Med Sci Sports Exerc 1998 (30) 4: 556 - 569

Fitzgerald GK; Open versus closed kinetic chain exercise: issues in rehabilitation after anterior cruciate reconstructive surgery. Phys Ther 1997 (77) 12: 1747 - 1754

Galtier B, Buillot M, Vanneuville G; Anatomical basis of the role of vastus medialis muscle in femoro-patellar degenerative arthropathy. Surg Radiol Anat 1995 (17) 1: 7 - 11

Garsden LR, Bullock-Saxton JE; Joint Reposition Sense in Subjects with Unilateral osteoarthritis of the Knee. Clin Rehabil 1999 (13) 2: 148 - 155

Gedalia U, Solomonow M, Zhou BH, Baratta RV, Lu Y, Harris M; Biomechanics of Increased Exposure to Lumbar Injury Caused by Cyclic Loading. Part 2. Recovery of Reflexive Muscular Stability With Rest. Spine 1999 (24) 23: 2461 - 2467

Grabiner MD, Koh TJ, Miller GF; Fatigue rates of vastus medialis oblique and vastus lateralis during statis and dynamic knee extension. J Orthop Res 1991 (9) 3: 391 - 397

Greenough CG, Oliver CW, Jones APC; Assessment of Spinal Musculature Using Surface Electromyographic Color Mapping. Spine 1998 (23) 16: 1768 - 1774

Goh JC, Lee PY, Bose K; A cadaver study of the function of the oblique part of vastus medialis. J Bone Joint Surgery 1995 (77) 2: 225 - 231

Hides JA, Richardson CA, Jull GA; Multifidus Muscle Recovery is Not Automatic After Resolution of Acute, First-Episode Low Back Pain. Spine 1996 (21) 23: 2763 - 2769

Hides JA, Stokes MJ, Saide M, Jull GA Cooper DH; Evidence of Lumbar Multifidus Muscle Wasting Ipsilateral to Symptoms in Patients with Acute/Subacute Low Back Pain. Spine 1994 (19) 2: 165 - 172

Hodges PW, Gandevia SC, Richardson CA; Contractions of Specific Abdominal Muscles in Postural Tasks are Affected by Respiratory Maneuvers. J Applied Physiol 1997 (83) 3: 753 - 760

Hodges PW, Richardson CA; Feedforward contraction of transversus abdominis is not influenced by arm movement. Exp Brain Res 1997 (114): 362 - 370

Hodges PW, Butler JE, McKenzie DK, Gandevia SC; Contraction of the human diaphragm during rapid postural adjustments. J of Physiology 1997 (505) 2: 539 - 548

Hodges PW, Richardson CA; Inefficient Muscular Stabilization of the Lumbar Spine Associated with Low Back Pain. A Motor Control Evaluation of Transversus Abdominis. Spine 1996 (21) 22: 2640 - 2650

Hodges PW, Richardson CA; The Influence of isometric hip adduction on quadriceps femoris activity. Scand J Rehabil Med 1993 (25) 2: 57 - 62

Hubbard JK, Sampson HW, Elledge JR; Prevalence and morphology of the vastus medialis oblique muscle in human cadavers. Anat Rec 1997 (249) 1: 135 - 142

Hubbard JK, Sampson HW, Elledge JR; The vastus medialis oblique muscle and its relationship to patellofemoral joint deterioration in human cadavers. J Orthop Sports Phys Ther 1998 (28) 6: 384 - 391

Karst GM, Willett GM; Onset timing of electromyographic activity in the vastus medialis oblique and vastus lateralis muscles in subjects with and without patellofemoral pain syndrome. Phys Ther 1995 (75) 9: 813 - 823

Klein BJ, Radeki RT, Foris MP, Feil EI, Hickey ME; Bridging the Gap Between Science and Practice in Managing Low Back Pain. Spine 2000 (25) 6: 738 - 740

Lieb FJ, Perry J; Quadriceps Function. J Bone Joint Surg 1968 (50-A) 8: 1535 - 1548

Liggett, CA; The Swiss Ball: An Overview of Applications in Sports Medicine. J Manual Manip Ther 1999 (7) 4: 190 - 196

Luoto S, Aalto H, Taimela S, Hurri H, Pyykko I, Alaranta H; One-Footed and Externally Disturbed Two-Footed Postural Control in Patients With Chronic Low Back Pain and Healthy Control Subjects. Spine 1998 (23) 19: 2081 - 2090

Lutz GE, Palmitier RA, An KN Chao EY; Comparison of tibiofemoral joint forces during open-kinetic-chain and closed-kinetic-chain exercises. 1993 (75) 5: 732 - 739

Lotz, JC, Colliou OK, Chin JR, Duncan NA, Libenberg E; Compression-Induced Degeneration of the Intervertebral Disc: An in vivo Mouse Model and Finite Element Study. Spine 1998 (23) 23: 2493 - 2506

MacIntosh JE, Bogduk N; The Attachments of the Lumbar Erector Spinae. Spine 1991 (16) 7: 783 - 792

Mannion AF, Muntener M, Taimela S, Dvorak J; A Randomized Clinical Trial of Three Active Therapies for Chronic Low Back Pain. Spine 1999 (24) 23: 2435 - 2448

Massion J; Movement, Posture and Equilibrium: Interaction and Coordination. Progress in Neurobiol 1992 (38): 35 - 56

McGill SM; Low Back Exercises: Evidence for Improving Exercise Regimens. Phys Ther 1998 (78): 754 - 765

McGill SM: Kinetic Potential of the Lumbar Trunk Musculature About Three Orthogonal Orthopaedic Axes in Extreme Postures. Spine 1991 (16) 7: 809 - 815

McLain RF; Mechanoreceptor Endings in Human Cervical Facet Joints. Spine (1994 919) 5: 495 - 501

Michelson JD, Hutchins C, Mechanoreceptors in the human ankle ligaments. J Bone Joint Surgery 1995 (77) 2: 219 - 224

Mirzabeigi E, Jordan C, Gronley JK, Rockowitz NL, Perry J; Isolation of the vastus medialis oblique muscle during exercise. Am J Sports Med 1999 (27) 1: 50 - 53

Mouchnino L, Aurenty R, Massion J, Pedotti A; Coordination Between Equilibrium and Head-Trunk Orientation During Leg Movement: A New Strategy Built Up by Training. J Neurophysiology 1992 (67) 6: 1587 - 1598

Norris CM; Spinal Stabilisation. Muscle Imbalance and the Low Back. Physiotherapy 1995 (81) 3: 127 - 138

Norris CM; Spinal Stabilisation. An Exercise Programme to Enhance Lumbar Stabilisation. Physiotherapy 1995 (81) 3: 138 - 146

Okawa A, Shinomiya K, Komori H, Muneta T, Arai Y, Nakai O; Dynamic Motion Study of the Whole Lumbar Spine by Videofluoroscopy. Spine 1998 (23) 16: 1743 - 1749

Oxland T, Panjabi MM; The Onset and Progression of Spinal Injury: A Demonstration of Neutral Zone Sensitivity. J Biomechanics 1992 (25) 10: 1165 - 1172
Panjabi MM, Kifune M, Liu W, Arand M, Vasavada A, Oxland TR; Graded thoracolumbar spinal injuries: development of multidirectional instability. Eur Spine J 1998 (7): 332 - 339

Panjabi MM; The Stabilizing System of the Spine. Part 1. Function, Dysfunction, Adaptation and Enhancement. J Spinal Disorders 1992 (5) 4: 383 - 389

Panjabi MM; The Stabilizing System of the Spine. Part 2. Neutral Zone and Instability Hypothesis. J Spinal Disorders 1992 (5) 4: 390 - 397

Panjabi MM; Experimental Determination of Spinal Motion Segment Behaviour. Ortho Clinics of North Am 1977 (8) 1: 169 - 180

Petrofsky JS, Phillips CA; Closed-loop control of movement of skeletal muscle. Crit Rev Biomed Eng 1985 (13) 1: 35 - 96

Pool-Goudzwaard AL, Vleeming A, Stoeckart R, Snijders CJ, Mens JMA; Insufficient lumbopelvic Stability: a clinical, anatomical and biomechanical approach to 'a-specific' low back pain. Manual Therapy 1998 (3) 1: 12 - 20

Quint U, Wilke HJ, Shirazi A, Parnianpour M, Loer F, Claes LE: Importance of the Intersegmental Trunk Muscles for the Stability of the Lumbar Spine. Spine 1998 (23) 18: 1937 - 1945

Radebold A, Cholewicki J, Panjabi MM, Patel TC; Muscle Response Pattern to Sudden Trunk Loading in Healthy Individuals and in Patients with Chronic Low Back Pain. Spine 2000 (25) 8: 947 - 954

Raimondo RA, Ahmad CS, Blankevoort L, April EW, Grelsamer RP, Henry JH; Patellar stabilization: a quantitative evaluation of the vastus medialis oblique muscle. Orthopedics 1998 (21) 7: 791 - 795

Rantanen J, Hurme M, Falck B, Alaranta H, Nykvist F, Lehto M, Einola S, Kalimo H; The Lumbar Multifidus Muscle Five Years After Surgery for a Lumbar Intervertebral Disc Herniation. Spine 1993 (18) 5: 568 - 574

Roberts S, Eisenstein SM, Menage J, Evans EH, Ashton IK; Mechanoreceptors in Intervertebral Discs. Morphology, distribution and Neuropeptides. Spine 1995 (20) 24: 2645 - 2651

Safran MR, Allen AA, Lephart SM, Borsa PA, Fu FH, Harner CD; Proprioception in the posterior cruciate ligament deficient knee. Knee Surg Sports Traumtol Arthrosc 1999 (7) 5: 310 - 317

Sato K, Kikuchi S, Yonezawa T; In Vivo Intradiscal Pressure Measurement in Healthy Individuals and in Patients With Ongoing Back Problems. Spine 1999 (24) 23: 2468 - 2474

Texts

Agur AMR, Ed; Grant's Atlas of Anatomy. Williams & Wilkins, 1991

Bogduk N; Clinical Anatomy of the Lumbar Spine and Sacrum, 3rd Ed. Churchill Livingstone, 1997

Grelsamer RP, McConnell J; The Patella. Aspen, 1998

Hall CM, Brody LT; Therapeutic Exercise. Moving Toward Function. Lippincott Williams & Wilkins, 1999

Kapandji IA; The Physiology of the Joints, Vol 3. 2nd Ed. Churchill Livingstone 1974

Kasman G; Course Notes: Surface EMG and Biofeedback in Physical Therapy. Self Published, 1997

Lee D; The Pelvic Girdle. An Approach to the Examination and Treatment of the Lumbo-Pelvic-Hip Region 2nd Ed. Churchill Livingstone, 1999

Lephart SM, Fu FH; Proprioception and Neuromuscular Control in Joint Stability. Human Kinetics, 2000

Lieber RL; Skeletal Muscle Structure and Function. Implications for Rehabilitation and Sports Medicine. Williams & Wilkins, 1992

Moore KL; Clinically Oriented Anatomy 2nd Ed. Williams & Wilkins, 1985

Richardson CA, Jull GA, Hodges PW, Hides J; Therapeutic Exercise for Spinal Segmental Stabilization in Low Back Pain. Churchill Livingstone, 1999

Robinson AJ, Snyder-Mackler, L; Clinical Electrophysiology. Electrotherapy and Electrophysiologic Testing. Williams & Wilkins, 1995

Winter DA; Biomechanics and Motor Control of Human Movement. John Wiley and Sons, 1990

Sheehy P, Burdett RG, Irrang JJ, VanSwearingen J; An electromyographic study of vastus medialis oblique and vastus lateralis activity while ascending and descending steps. J Orthop Sports Phys Ther 1998 (27) 6: 423 - 429

Snook SH, Webster BS, McGorry RW, Fogleman MT, McCann KB; The Reduction of Chronic Nonspecific Low Back Pain Through the Control of Early Morning Lumbar Flexion. Spine 1998 (23) 23: 2601 - 2607

Solomonow M, Zhou B, Baratta RV, Lu Y, Harris M; Biomechanics of Increased Exposure to Lumbar Injury Caused by Cyclic Loading: Part 1. Loss of Reflexive Muscular Stabilization. Spine 1999 (24) 23: 2426 - 2434

Solomonow M, Zhou B, Harris M, Lu Y, Baratta RV; The Ligamento-Muscular Stabilizing System of the Spine. Spine 1998 (23) 23: 2552 - 2562

Solomonow M, Guanche C, Wink C, Knatt T, Baratta RV, Lu Y; Mechanoreceptors and reflex arc in the feline shoulder. J Shoulder Elbow Surg 1996 (5) 2: 139 - 146

Spencer JD, Hayes K, Alexander IJ; Knee Joint Effusion and Quadriceps Reflex Inhibition in Man. Arch Phys Med Rehabil 1984 (65): 171 - 177
Thiranagama R; Nerve Supply of the Human Vastus Medialis Muscle. J Anatomy 1990 (170): 193 - 198

Taimela S, Takala EP, Asklof T, Seppala K, Parviainen S; Active Treatment of Chronic Neck Pain. Spine 2000 (25) 8: 1021 - 1027

Valeriani M, Restuccia D, Di Lazzaro V, Franceschi F, Fabbriciani C, Tonali P; Clinical and Neuro-physiological Abnormalities Before and After Reconstruction of the Anterior Cruciate Ligament of the Knee. Acta Neurol Scand 1999 (99) 5: 303 - 307

Vangsness CT, Ennis M, Taylor JG, Atkinson R; Neural Anatomy of the Glenohumeral Ligaments, Labrum and Subacromial Bursa. Arthroscopy 1995 (11) 2: 180 - 184

Vernazza-Martin S, Martin N, Cincera M, Pedotti A, Massion J; Arm raising in humans under loaded vs. unloaded and bipedal vs. unipedal conditions. Brain Research 1999 (846): 12 - 22

Vezina MJ, Hubley-Kozey CL, Egan DA; A Review of the Muscle Activation Patterns Associated with the Pelvic Tilt Exercise Used in the Treatment of Low Back Pain. J Manual Manip Ther 1998 (6) 4: 191 - 201

Wilke HJ, Wolf S, Claes LE, Arand M, Wiesend A; Stability Increase of the Lumbar Spine With Different Muscle Groups. Spine 1995 (20) 2: 192 - 198

Wolf SL, Segal RL, English AW; Task-Oriented EMG Activity Recorded from Partitions in Human Lateral Gastrocnemius Muscle. J Electromyography Kinesiology 1993 (3) 2: 87 - 94

Zakaria D, Harburn KL, Kramer JF; Preferntial activation of the vastus medialis oblique, vastus lateralis, and hip adductor muscles during isometric exercises in females. J Orthop Sports Phys Ther 1997 (26) 1: 23 - 28